# TRACEY-LEE HOGAN

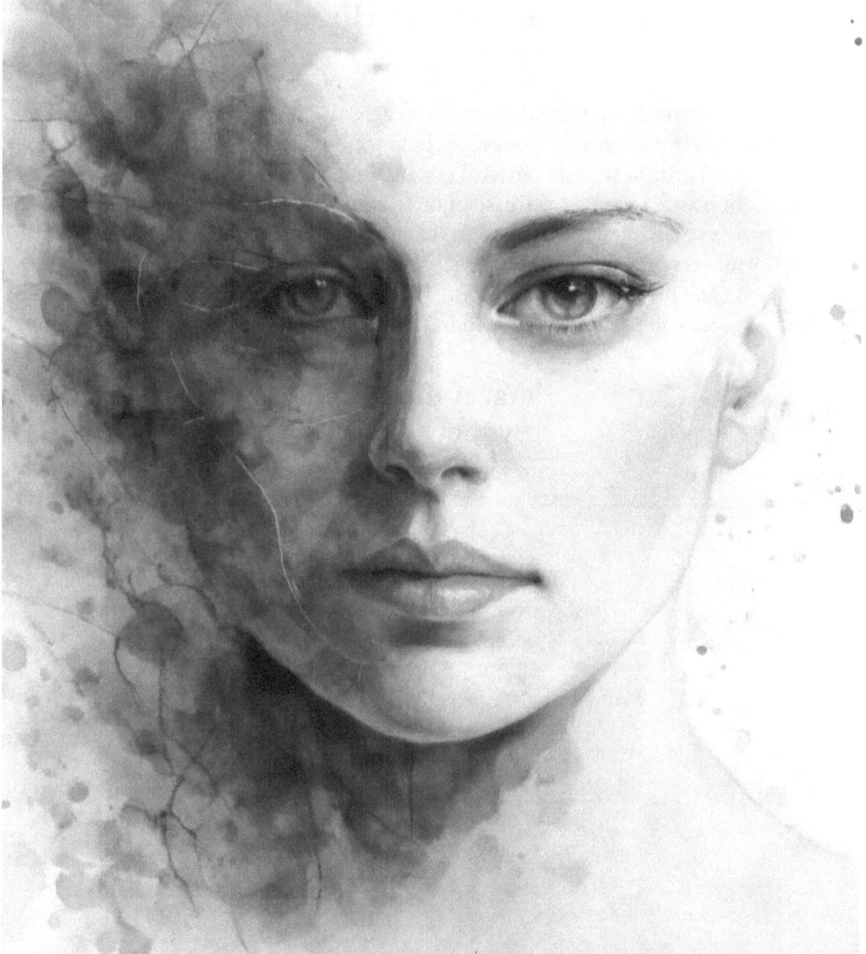

# LIFE AFTER NARCISSISTS
### IT'S TIME TO BE *happy* AGAIN

Copyright © 2025 by **Tracey-Lee Hogan**

All rights reserved. No part of this book may be used or reproduced by any means, graphic, electronic, or mechanical, including photocopying, recording, taping or by any information storage retrieval system without the written permission of the copyright owner except in the case of brief quotations embodied in critical articles and reviews. The views expressed in this work are solely those of the author and do not necessarily reflect the views of the publisher and the publisher hereby disclaims any responsibility for them. The author and publisher have taken steps to ensure that all parties mentioned in this book are protected from such threats.

**Tracey-Lee Hogan**
**Sydney, Australia**
lifeafternarcissists.com

Book Layout © Annie Gibbins
Book Cover design © Tracey-Lee Hogan
Proofreader @ Annie Gibbins
Editor @ Prudence Clark
Professional Photo @ imagesbysophie.com.au

ISBN 978-1-922969-30-9

*Women's Biz*
**Global**

## Legal Disclaimer and Scope

This book is a work of non-fiction that combines personal narrative, professional reflection, and discussion of publicly available research across psychology, trauma studies, stress physiology, attachment theory, and complementary medicine. It is provided for **educational and informational purposes only**. Nothing in this book constitutes medical, psychological, psychiatric, legal, or other professional advice, nor is it intended to substitute for individual assessment, diagnosis, or care by a qualified professional. Readers are encouraged to seek appropriate professional support relevant to their circumstances. Personal narrative sections reflect the author's lived experience and perspective. Any clinical examples, workplace scenarios, or relationship descriptions are **composite, de-identified, and fictionalised**, constructed from recurring patterns observed across multiple individuals over time. These composites are illustrative only and do not represent or refer to any specific real person, living or deceased. Any resemblance to actual persons, events, or situations is coincidental.

References to interpersonal dynamics, behavioural patterns, or traits (including descriptions sometimes referred to as "narcissistic traits") are used **descriptively and non-diagnostically**. No individual is identified, assessed, or diagnosed within this work, and no mental disorder is attributed to any person. Behavioural descriptions should not be interpreted as psychiatric classification.

Scientific and clinical information discussed is grounded in peer-reviewed research and recognised theoretical models. Where explanatory frameworks are referenced (including, but not limited to, attachment theory, stress physiology, or autonomic regulation models), they are presented as **interpretive frameworks** rather than definitive, exhaustive, or universally accepted mechanisms. Statements describing physiological or psychological responses reflect tendencies and adaptations reported in the literature, not deterministic or guaranteed outcomes.

The author and publisher make no representations or warranties regarding the accuracy, completeness, applicability, or suitability of the information for any particular individual or purpose. To the maximum extent permitted by applicable law, the author and publisher disclaim liability for any loss, harm, or damages arising directly or indirectly from the use, interpretation, or reliance upon the material in this book. Nothing in this disclaimer is intended to exclude rights that cannot be excluded under applicable consumer protection laws.

This book is not intended to accuse, identify, or characterise any individual or organisation, nor to allege wrongdoing by any identifiable person. Interpretations drawn by readers are their own and are not asserted or endorsed by the author.

# CONTENTS

DEDICATION ................................................................ 22
CHAPTER ONE ........................................................... 26
Childhood, Fear, and Survival Patterns ................................ 26
   The House of Chaos and Silence ..................................... 26
   Reflections ............................................................... 33
CHAPTER TWO ........................................................... 36
Learning to Hide in Plain Sight ........................................ 36
   Reflections ............................................................... 41
CHAPTER THREE ....................................................... 43
Relationship Dynamics ................................................. 43
   Angela - Choosing Stability that Looked Like Safety ........... 44
   Rachael - When "Practical" Quietly Became Conditional ....... 47
   Nicole - When the Body Ends the Conversation ................. 50
   Poppy - Pregnancy, Vulnerability and Emotional Absence ..... 52
   Eloise - Illness without Support ...................................... 54
   Jennifer - The Exit Begins in the Body ............................ 56
   Letisha - Aftermath – When a Relationship is Over, is it Really? ... 58
   Claire - Aftermath, When a Pet Becomes a Pawn ............... 60
   Reflections ............................................................... 63
CHAPTER FOUR .......................................................... 67
Work – The Final Bastion .............................................. 67
   Part I ..................................................................... 67
   Part II .................................................................... 69
   Part III ................................................................... 73
   Work Collaboration: the opposite experience. .................... 73
   Reflections ............................................................... 76
CHAPTER FIVE ........................................................... 79

The Apex Break ................................................................................. 79
    Reflections ................................................................................ 83
CHAPTER SIX ............................................................................... 85
Stabilisation and Insight ............................................................... 85
    Reflections ................................................................................ 87
CHAPTER SEVEN ........................................................................ 90
Integration and Peace .................................................................. 90
    Reflections ................................................................................ 93
CHAPTER EIGHT ......................................................................... 96
From My Experience to Your Clarity ........................................... 96
PART II ........................................................................................... 99
CHAPTER NINE ......................................................................... 100
Understanding Narcissistic Behaviour Types and How They Present During Interactions with You ..................................................... 100
Narcissistic Supply ..................................................................... 102
Future Faking ............................................................................. 104
    Word Salad, or Circular Conversations ................................. 107
    Triangulation .......................................................................... 108
    D.A.R.V.O. ............................................................................. 108
Stage 3: Discard or Withdrawal ................................................. 109
    Reactive Abuse ...................................................................... 111
    9.2 Types of Narcissistic Behaviour ...................................... 113
    Grandiose Narcissism ............................................................ 113
    Vulnerable (Covert) Narcissism ............................................. 114
    Communal (Benevolent) Narcissism ..................................... 118
    Client Example ....................................................................... 119
Why this Example Fits Communal Narcissistic Behaviour ....... 120
Malignant Behaviour Patterns ................................................... 122
    Key Features in the Research ............................................... 122
Examples ..................................................................................... 123

Machiavellian Behaviour ... 125
Research-Based Example of Machiavellian Behaviour ... 128
   References (for the example above) ... 129
9.3 Why People Feel So Confused After Experiencing Narcissistic Behaviours ... 130
Why the Nervous System Struggles to Make Sense of Narcissistic Abuse ... 130
Why Narcissistic Abuse Feels So Personal - But Isn't ... 131
CHAPTER TEN ... 133
Behaviour Clusters that Destabilise ... 133
10.1 - Behaviour Cluster Overview ... 133
10.1.1 - Bonding Behaviours ... 134
   Love Bombing ... 134
   Future Faking ... 134
10.1.2 - Destabilisation Behaviours ... 135
   Gaslighting ... 135
   Word Salad ... 135
   Triangulation ... 135
   Circular Conversations ... 136
10.1.3 - Control Behaviours ... 136
   Devaluation ... 136
   DARVO ... 136
10.1.4 - Exit Behaviours ... 137
   Hoovering ... 137
Why These Behaviours Create Confusion ... 137
Integration of Behaviour Clusters ... 138
CHAPTER ELEVEN ... 139
The Disengagement: When the Pattern Ends Abruptly ... 139
   1. Abrupt Relational Rupture as a Stressor ... 139
   2. Loss of Predictability and the Brain's Response ... 140
   3. Cognitive Dissonance During Abrupt Disengagement ... 141

    4. Shame as a Neurobiological Response ............................................ 141
    5. Allostatic Load and the "Final Stressor" Concept ......................... 142
    6. The Sudden Silence: Why the Nervous System Reacts ................. 142
    7. Documented Emotional and Physical Reactions ............................ 143
    8. Why Understanding the Physiology Helps ..................................... 143
CHAPTER TWELVE .................................................................................. 145
Why Clarity Comes After Distance ........................................................... 145
    1. Distance Lets Your Nervous System Settle ...................................... 145
    2. Your Cognitive Bandwidth Returns .................................................. 146
    3. Your Internal Cues Reappear ............................................................. 146
    4. The Cognitive Dissonance Reduces ................................................... 147
    5. Safety Allows Accurate Perspective .................................................. 147
    6. Insight Is No Longer Interrupted ...................................................... 148
    7. Why You Didn't See It Earlier ........................................................... 148
    8. Your System Begins to Regulate ........................................................ 149
    Reflections ................................................................................................. 150
    1. The Nervous System Needs Safety Before Insight is Possible ..... 150
    2. Cognitive Load Reduces and Processing Returns ......................... 150
    3. Internal Cues Re-Activate When External Pressure Stops .......... 151
    4. Reduced Exposure Means Reduced Dissonance ........................... 151
    5. Safety Restores Perspective ................................................................ 152
    6. Integration is a Physiological Response, Not a Moral One ......... 152
CHAPTER THIRTEEN ............................................................................... 154
The Stabilisation Phase ................................................................................ 154
1. Physiological Stabilisation ..................................................................... 154
    1.1 The threat response begins to stand down ................................... 154
    1.2 Cortisol begins to regulate ............................................................... 155
    1.3 Digestion reawakens ......................................................................... 155
    1.4 Sleep recalibrates – Gradually ......................................................... 156
    1.5 Clarity windows appear - Then fade ............................................. 156

2. Emotional Stabilisation .................................................................. 156
    2.1 Emotional flattening is a normal transition ............................... 157
    2.2 Delayed emotions are expected .................................................. 157
    2.3 The system may not register calm as familiar ............................ 157
    2.4 Relief and loneliness can coexist ................................................ 157
    2.5 The relationship comes into focus ............................................. 158
    2.6 Instinct begins to return ............................................................. 158
The Further You Distance Yourself ...................................................... 159
    1. Cognitive Load Reduces Before Insight Appears ....................... 159
    2. Processing Capacity Changes - Including Micro-Cognition ........ 160
    3. Emotional and Cognitive Systems Come Back Online Out of Sync
    ................................................................................................................ 161
    4. Memory Integration Improves Without Active Effort ............... 161
    5. Recognition Replaces Confusion ................................................ 162
    6. The Smoke and Mirrors Fall Away .............................................. 162
    7. Clarity Is a Physiological Process ................................................ 163
What Recovery Isn't ............................................................................... 163
    1. Recovery is not instantaneous clarity ......................................... 164
    2. Recovery is not emotional catharsis .......................................... 164
    3. Recovery is not a "positive mindset" process ............................ 164
    4. Recovery is not linear .................................................................. 165
    5. Recovery is not immediate self-trust ......................................... 165
    6. Recovery is not emotional independence ................................. 166
    7. Recovery is not an identity shift ................................................ 166
    8. Recovery is not quick .................................................................. 166
    9. Recovery is not a moral test ....................................................... 167
    10. Recovery is not a diagnosis of the other person ..................... 167
Relearning Your Baseline ....................................................................... 168
1. Recalibration After Chronic Stress .................................................... 168
2. Rediscovering Preferences and Needs .............................................. 169

3. Recognising Internal Signals Again ........................................................ 169
4. Choosing Support that Supports You .................................................... 170
5. Why Relational Clarity Takes Time ....................................................... 171
6. Building Slowly, Not Dramatically ........................................................ 171
Relearning Your Baseline, Part II ................................................................ 172
1. Your Capacity Expands in Small, Measurable Ways ........................... 172
2. Social Filters Improve ............................................................................. 173
3. Daily Life Becomes Simpler (which is a milestone, not a regression) ........................................................................................................................... 173
4. You Start to Rebuild Your Internal Sense of Safety ............................ 174
5. If You Are Not Able to Leave Your Situation Yet ............................... 175
6. Steady Doesn't Mean Finished ............................................................... 175
The First Signs of Reconnection ................................................................. 176
   1. Curiosity Returns in Small, Manageable Pieces ............................. 176
   2. Your Internal Pace Evens Out ............................................................ 177
   3. Preferences Start Returning ............................................................... 177
   4. Your Capacity for Connection With Others Changes .................. 177
   5. Your Sense of Humour Shifts ............................................................ 178
   6. You Notice Small Threads of Future Thinking .............................. 178
   7. Your Body Begins to Trust You Again ............................................ 179
   8. You Begin to Look at Your Story Without Overwhelm ............... 179
PART III .......................................................................................................... 181
CHAPTER FOURTEEN ............................................................................. 182
The Hogan Method: What it is and isn't .................................................. 182
   1. Why This Method Exists .................................................................... 183
   2. What the Method *Is* .......................................................................... 184
   3. What the Method *Isn't* ..................................................................... 184
   4. Why Body Recovery Matters ............................................................. 185
   5. What You Can Expect From This Section ...................................... 185
   6. A Note Before We Begin .................................................................... 186

Early Physical Changes in Stabilisation ........................................................ 186
   1. Breathing Becomes Less Shallow ................................................. 187
   2. Muscle Tension Begins to Ease..................................................... 187
   3. Energy Levels Begin to Stabilise .................................................. 188
   4. Digestive Function starts to settle ............................................... 188
   5. Sleep Begins to Shift .................................................................... 188
   6. The Immune System Responds More Appropriately.................. 189
   7. Headaches, Migraines and Sensory Sensitivity Can Improve ...... 190
When Cognitive Function Begins to Return ................................................. 190
   1. Executive Functioning Improves in Small, Practical Ways ......... 190
   2. Micro-Cognition Starts to Stabilise.............................................. 191
   3. The Capacity for Perspective-Taking Expands............................ 191
   4. Emotional Reasoning and Catastrophising Reduce .................... 192
   5. Attention Capacity Improves ...................................................... 192
   6. The Ability to Make Decisions Reappears.................................. 193
   7. Retrospective Clarity Increases ................................................... 193
   Example - A Woman Balancing Work and Young Children .......... 195
   8. Why High-Functioning People Often Experience Delayed Cognitive Return ............................................................................. 196
   9. A Note on Expectations .............................................................. 196
CHAPTER FIFTEEN .................................................................................... 197
The Naturopathic Bridge ............................................................................... 197
15.1 - Nervous System Nutrients................................................................... 199
Magnesium..................................................................................................... 200
Thiamine (Vitamin B1) ................................................................................. 201
Riboflavin (VitaminB2)................................................................................. 202
Niacin (Vitamin B3) ...................................................................................... 203
Pantothenic Acid (Vitamin B5) ..................................................................... 204
Pyridoxine (Vitamin B6)................................................................................ 204
Folate (Vitamin B9) ....................................................................................... 205

Methylfolate ..................................................................................................206

Cobalamin (Vitamin B12) ................................................................................207

Choline ...........................................................................................................207

Inositol ...........................................................................................................208

1. What it does ...............................................................................................208

15.2 - Energy Nutrients ..................................................................................209

1. B Vitamins - The Core Energy Group ........................................................209

    1.1 Vitamin B1 (Thiamine) ........................................................................209

    1.2 Vitamin B2 (Riboflavin).......................................................................210

    1.3 Vitamin B3 (Niacin) ............................................................................211

    1.4 Vitamin B5 (Pantothenic Acid) ............................................................212

    1.5 Vitamin B6 (Pyridoxine) .....................................................................213

    1.6 Vitamin B12 (Cobalamin) ...................................................................213

    1.7 Folate (Vitamin B9) ............................................................................214

    1.8 Iron ....................................................................................................215

2. Additional Energy-Supporting Nutrients ....................................................216

    2.1 Magnesium ........................................................................................216

    2.2 Iodine .................................................................................................216

    2.3 Selenium ............................................................................................217

    2.4 Chromium .........................................................................................217

    2.5 Inositol ...............................................................................................217

15.3 — Sleep Support Nutrients .....................................................................218

1. Magnesium .................................................................................................218

2. Calcium ......................................................................................................219

3. Vitamin D ..................................................................................................220

4. Vitamin B6 .................................................................................................221

5. Zinc ............................................................................................................221

6. Iron ............................................................................................................222

15.4 - Digestive Support Nutrients .................................................................223

1. B Vitamins - Supporting Energy, Nerve Signalling and Cell Repair.224

2. Vitamin D - Immune Modulation and Gut Barrier Support ............ 225
3. Zinc - Repairing Gut Tissue and Supporting Immune Function ...... 226
4. Vitamin E - Antioxidant Support for Gut Tissue ............................... 227
5. Probiotics ........................................................................................... 228
A Note on Stress and Digestive Symptoms ............................................ 228
15.5 - Herbal Medicines for Nervous System Stability ......................... 229
    What it does .................................................................................... 230
    Why it helps under stress ................................................................ 231
    Symptoms that may shift ................................................................ 231
    Cross-system overlap ...................................................................... 231
    Clinician note. ................................................................................. 231
    References ....................................................................................... 232
2. *Lavandula angustifolia* (Lavender — Herb and Essential Oil) ............ 232
    What it does .................................................................................... 232
    Why it helps under stress ................................................................ 232
    Symptoms that may shift ................................................................ 232
    Cross-system overlap ...................................................................... 233
    Clinician note. ................................................................................. 233
    References ....................................................................................... 233
3. *Melissa officinalis* (Lemon Balm) ...................................................... 233
    What it does .................................................................................... 233
    Why it helps under stress ................................................................ 234
    Symptoms that may shift ................................................................ 234
    Cross-system overlap ...................................................................... 234
    Clinician note. ................................................................................. 234
    References ....................................................................................... 234
4. *Passiflora incarnata* (Passionflower) ................................................. 235
    What it does .................................................................................... 235
    Why it helps under stress ................................................................ 235
    Symptoms that may shift ................................................................ 235

  Cross-system overlap ...................................................................235
  Clinician note ..............................................................................235
  References ...................................................................................235
5. *Scutellaria lateriflora* (Skullcap) ....................................................236
  What it does ................................................................................236
  Why it helps under stress ..........................................................236
  Cross-system overlap ...................................................................236
  Clinician note ..............................................................................236
  References ...................................................................................236
6. *Leonurus cardiaca* (Motherwort) ...................................................237
  What it does ................................................................................237
  Why it helps under stress ..........................................................237
  Symptoms that may shift............................................................237
  Cross-system overlap ...................................................................237
  Clinician note ..............................................................................237
  References ...................................................................................237
  SECTION 1B - Adaptogens ......................................................238
1. *Withania somnifera* (Ashwagandha)................................................238
  What it does................................................................................238
  Why it helps under chronic stress ............................................239
  Symptoms that may shift............................................................239
  Cross-system overlap ...................................................................239
  Clinician note ..............................................................................239
  References ...................................................................................239
2. *Schisandra chinensis* (Schisandra).....................................................240
  What it does ................................................................................240
  Why it helps under chronic stress ............................................240
  Symptoms that may shift............................................................240
  Cross-system overlap ...................................................................240
  Clinician note ..............................................................................241

References ............................................................................. 241

3. *Ocimum tenuiflorum / O. sanctum* (Holy Basil / Tulsi) ........................ 241

    What it does ........................................................................ 241

    Cross-system overlap ........................................................... 242

    Clinician note ...................................................................... 242

    References ........................................................................... 242

4. *Bacopa monnieri* (Bacopa) ............................................................ 242

    What it does ........................................................................ 242

    Symptoms that may shift .................................................... 243

    Cross-system overlap ........................................................... 243

    Clinician note ...................................................................... 243

    References ........................................................................... 243

5. *Crocus sativus* (Saffron) ............................................................... 243

    What it does ........................................................................ 244

    Why it helps under chronic stress ...................................... 244

    Cross-system overlap ........................................................... 244

    Clinician note ...................................................................... 244

    References ........................................................................... 244

    SECTION 1C – Multifunctional Nervous System Herbs ............. 245

1. *Ziziphus jujuba var. spinosa* (Zizyphus) ....................................... 245

    What it does ........................................................................ 245

    Clinician note ...................................................................... 245

    References ........................................................................... 246

2. *Valeriana officinalis* (Valerian) .................................................... 246

    What it does ........................................................................ 246

    Symptoms that may shift .................................................... 246

    Cross-system overlap ........................................................... 247

    Clinician note ...................................................................... 247

    References ........................................................................... 247

3. *Eschscholzia californica* (California poppy) .................................. 247

What it does ...................................................................................248

Cross-system overlap ....................................................248

Clinician note. ..................................................................248

References ........................................................................248

SECTION 1D - Sleep Focused Herbs .........................249

1. *Passiflora incarnata* (Passionflower) ...............................249

What it does ...................................................................249

Why it helps under chronic stress ................................249

Symptoms that may shift ..............................................250

Cross-system overlap ....................................................250

References ........................................................................250

3. *Melissa officinalis* (Lemon balm) ....................................250

What it does ...................................................................251

Why it helps under chronic stress ................................251

Cross-system overlap ....................................................251

References ........................................................................252

Immune–Stress Adaptation Herbs ........................................252

1 *Eleutherococcus senticosus* (Siberian ginseng /Eleuthero) .........252

2 *Echinacea* spp. (Echinacea) .............................................253

3 *Ocimum tenuiflorum* / *O. sanctum* (Holy basil / Tulsi) ..........254

4 *Schisandra chinensis* (Schisandra) ..................................255

5 *Albizia lebbeck* (Albizia) ..................................................255

6 *Uncaria tomentosa* (Cat's claw) ......................................257

7 *Hericium erinaceus* (Lion's mane mushroom) ..............257

SECTION 2 - Digestive Herbs ................................................259

*Matricaria chamomilla* / *Matricaria recutita* (German Chamomile) ........259

*Zingiber officinale* (Ginger) ...........................................261

*Mentha* × *piperita* (Peppermint) .........................................262

*Foeniculum vulgare* (Fennel) ...............................................264

*Cynara scolymus* (Globe artichoke) ....................................265

*Ulmus rubra* (Slippery elm) .................................................................. 267
15.6 - Pain and Inflammation Herbs ......................................................... 269
   Introduction ........................................................................................ 269
Why Stress Increases Inflammatory Mediators ........................................ 269
How Inflammation Drives Chronic Pain ................................................. 270
When Stress is Ongoing and Inflammatory Mediators Stay Elevated .. 270
1. *Curcuma longa* (Turmeric / Curcumin) ............................................. 270
2. *Boswellia serrata* ................................................................................ 272
3. *Harpagophytum procumbens* (Devil's Claw) ..................................... 273
4. *Salix alba* (White Willow Bark) ......................................................... 274
5. *Zingiber officinale* (Ginger) ................................................................ 275
CHAPTER 15.7 - Other Supplements: A Special Mention .................... 277
1. Coenzyme Q10 (CoQ10 / Ubiquinone / Ubiquinol) ........................ 277
2. Omega-3 Fatty Acids (EPA & DHA) ................................................. 279
3. Glutamine (L-Glutamine) .................................................................. 280
4. L-Theanine ......................................................................................... 281
5. Lactoferrin .......................................................................................... 282
15.8 - Dietary Choices: Feeding Your Body ............................................ 283
1. Foods and Substances to Reduce ...................................................... 283
   1.1 Alcohol ......................................................................................... 284
   1.2 Caffeine ........................................................................................ 284
   1.3 Ultra-processed foods, artificial additives, and preservatives .... 284
   1.4 Fast food and packaged convenience foods ............................. 285
2. Foods to Prioritise .............................................................................. 285
   2.1 Fresh vegetables and fruits .......................................................... 285
   2.2 Whole grains ................................................................................ 286
   2.3 Quality protein sources ............................................................... 286
   2.4 Avoid processed meats ................................................................ 286
   2.5 Fresh vegetable juices .................................................................. 286
3. A Practical Naturopathic Framework ................................................ 287

## 15.9 - Movement and Lifestyle Fundamentals ............................. 287
### 1. Why Movement Matters in Recovery ..................................... 288
### 2. Practical Movement Options (Evidence-Based) ..................... 288
#### 2.1 Walking ................................................................................ 289
#### 2.2 Gentle Strength Work ............................................................ 289
#### 2.3 Yoga (Evidence-Based) .......................................................... 289
#### 2.4 Stretching and Mobility Work ............................................... 290
#### 2.5 Nature Exposure (Green Exercise) ....................................... 290
### 3. Supporting Lifestyle Practices .............................................. 291
#### 3.1 Regularity of sleep and waking times .................................. 291
#### 3.2 Morning light exposure ......................................................... 291
#### 3.3 Reduced sensory load ........................................................... 291
#### 3.4 Social contact that is predictable and low-pressure ............ 291
## 15.10 - Environmental Stabilisation (Your Home as a Healing Space) 292
### 1. Why Your Environment Matters in Recovery ........................ 292
### 2. Predictability: The Foundation of Environmental Stabilisation ........ 293
### 3. Light, Air, and Sensory Load .................................................. 294
#### 3.1 Light ....................................................................................... 294
#### 3.2 Air .......................................................................................... 294
#### 3.3 Sensory Load ......................................................................... 294
### 4. Creating Micro-Zones of Support ........................................... 295
#### 4.1 A Calm Corner ...................................................................... 295
#### 4.2 A Sleep-Protective Zone ....................................................... 295
#### 4.3 A Clarity Zone ...................................................................... 296
### 5. Natural Elements ..................................................................... 296
### 6. Reducing Environmental Triggers ........................................ 297
## 15.11 Building Predictable Routines ........................................... 297
### Why Predictability Matters ......................................................... 298
### 2. Routine as a Biological Cue .................................................... 298
### 3. Start Small: Micro-Routines .................................................... 299

4. Why Routines Feel Different After Stress ............................................... 299
5. The Role of External Supports ................................................................ 300
6. Anchor Points: The Non-Negotiable Few ............................................... 300
CHAPTER SIXTEEN ..................................................................................... 302
Pulling it All Together With the Hogan Method ....................................... 302
1. The Hogan Method Approach ................................................................ 302
2. What the Hogan Method Is Not ............................................................. 303
3. Why the Method Works in Stages ......................................................... 304
4. Core Pillars of the Hogan Method ......................................................... 305
   Pillar 1 - Clarity Through Education ..................................................... 305
   Pillar 2 - Nervous System Support ........................................................ 305
   Pillar 3 - Digestive and Immune Restoration ....................................... 305
   Pillar 4 - Sleep Recalibration ................................................................. 305
   Pillar 5 - Inflammation and Pain Support ............................................ 305
   Pillar 6 - Thoughtful Supplementation ................................................. 305
   Pillar 7 - Lifestyle Anchors ..................................................................... 305
   Pillar 8 - Reconnection With Self .......................................................... 306
5. When to Seek Professional Support ...................................................... 306
6. Where You Go From Here ...................................................................... 306
7. A Final Note from Me .............................................................................. 307
CHAPTER REFERENCES ............................................................................. 309
Chapters 1, 2, and 3 ..................................................................................... 309
Chapter 4 References .................................................................................. 311
Chapter 5 References .................................................................................. 312
Chapter 6 References .................................................................................. 313
Chapter 7 References .................................................................................. 313
Chapter 8 – no references listed. ............................................................... 314
Chapter 9 References .................................................................................. 314
Chapter 10 References ................................................................................ 320
Chapter 11 References ................................................................................ 321

Chapter 12 References ..................................................................... 322
Chapter 13.1 References .................................................................. 323
Chapter 13.2 References .................................................................. 324
Chapter 13.3 References .................................................................. 324
Chapter 13.4 References .................................................................. 325
Chapter 13.5 References .................................................................. 326
Chapter 13.6 References .................................................................. 326
Chapter 14.2 References .................................................................. 327
Chapter 14.3 References .................................................................. 328
Chapter 15.1 References .................................................................. 329
Chapter 15.2 (Energy Nutrients) References ................................. 330
   B Vitamins ................................................................................... 330
   Minerals and Other Energy Nutrients ..................................... 332
Chapter 15.3 References .................................................................. 333
Chapter 15.4 References .................................................................. 334
Chapter 15.8 References .................................................................. 335
Chapter 15.9 References .................................................................. 336
Chapter 15.10 References ................................................................ 337
Chapter 15.11 References ................................................................ 338
FURTHER READING ................................................................... 340
ABOUT THE AUTHOR ................................................................ 346

## DEDICATION

I dedicate this book to all of the women who have walked through this; may you shine brightly once again.

Dear you,

Welcome to this book with open arms and a big hug from me.

You've more than likely arrived here because you, or someone you know or love, is at the point where you or they've been subjected to narcissistic behaviours.

You are looking for answers.

You are looking for the why.

You are looking for a way out, a way up, a way home to yourself. It's my hope that my story and this book resonate with you, and with that resonation you find comfort in knowing you aren't alone. It might seem that way now, but please know, there are people that can help you. There are many of us that have battled in a similar way, and yes, it's exhausting.

Becoming aligned with the research and knowledge is a good starting point, because once you see the patterns, you can't unsee them. It's helps you realise it's not you and never was.

My wish for you is that you reignite the bright shining spark in you, the playful, luminous, shining spark that might have been diminished for a time.

It's still there, and it's time to coax and stoke that spark back into a bright flame. When you are a light, you attract a lot of moths, so hopefully this book gives you the chance to recognise know just who those moths are and tell them to fuck off when the need arises. Metaphorically speaking.

May your light shine brightly on the world.

This book is quite the journey, because the first part is my own personal story. It's raw, true, and it's my earlier life. I've walked the planet now for over sixty years, so I've given up being scared to share it, in the hope it helps you.

The second part of the book is what I learnt over many years about abuse from a real, evidence-based approach to what happened, to not only me (which provided me with answers), but anyone else who has experienced abuse. There are distinct patterns, and it's almost like there's a playbook that people exhibiting these behaviours and traits work from.

It's important that you understand what the research is regarding these types of situations, so you can make decisions about what you, or someone you know, has experienced.

The third part of the book, based on recovery, is my wheelhouse. This is my special area of interest, and I hope it helps you, or your person, to recover, just as I have.

One thing I say to you, if it's not you, I will ask one thing. Please don't say to the person you are reading this for, "Why didn't you leave?" It's not helpful, because it's very complex, and this will become apparent as you read on….

If you are reading this for yourself, well done. You are braver than you know. You might not realise it now, but there will come a time when you settle into your bravery, so your light shines brightly again. This book is written for you.

With Grace and Love,

Tracey x

# PART 1
# Early Years and Foundations

# CHAPTER ONE

# Childhood, Fear, and Survival Patterns

**The House of Chaos and Silence**

My first memory occurs around two years of age. I'm wearing a blue jumper my gran had knitted me, and I'm eating cornflakes at her dining table because we were living with her at the time. My mother had a friend over, and the friend's daughter bites my shoulder so hard it makes me scream.

Mum says, "She didn't mean it, now go and play."

It was the first lesson in family- don't make a fuss about pain. It was the 1960's and you walked off everything, from sprains to concussions, back then. With no whining; it's what everyone did.

My next memory is when my father arrived home from the Vietnam War.

He knocked on the door and has arrived with gifts -a huge stuffed panda bear for Mum, a geisha doll in a plastic box, and a blue fluffy toy dog, that's also a radio for me, which I loved. I'm four years old and we had also just welcomed a baby sister into our family. I think he gifted her with a white fluffy dog radio as well. She was a newborn, so I think he might have thought she'd grow into loving it.

While Mum goes out to get some food, he questions me: What men has your mother been seeing?

I said "no-one". He keeps asking me, and I don't know any men, so I say the only name I can think of-Brian. My father asks what he looks like, and I told him he had brown hair and glasses.

"Brian", was Brian Henderson, the newsreader on television. He was in the living room every night, talking about the moon landing on the screen. He was the only man I knew besides my dad and my uncle.

After the ensuing screaming match between my mother and father, in a moment of rage and overwhelm, mum hit me across the legs with a hairbrush until it snapped. I don't write this to punish her. I write it to show how unsafe everything already was for all of us, and this was 1969. It was the time where children were smacked as a form of discipline, and being whipped across the hands, knuckles, or the back of the legs with a cane was a regular occurrence in schools.

From then on, I learnt that peace depended on being a good girl. Never mind the interrogation from the adult that forced me to find a male, any male, that my mother had apparently been seeing behind his back. I had simply wanted to answer my father's repeated question that he kept asking… remember I was four. From that moment on, I was always trying to be the perfect child for my mum.

On reflection, television was both a good babysitter, and distraction for me. Each morning, I watched Swami Sarasvati doing yoga, and I copied her movements on the lounge-room floor. My tiny body was learning yoga poses, stretching, breathing, and I really thought it was fun. It was unknowingly the first nervous-system regulation I ever practised.

We moved out of where we were living with my gran, and from then on, we'd have to move often. We lived in Manly for a short while, then to the house across from my father's mechanical workshop in Freshwater. That's where I first remembered seeing the horrific violence between my mum and father. He king-hit mum in broad daylight, while she was holding my baby sister. I remember running down the street screaming: Call the police!

A couple from a nearby house pulled me inside and hid me until the sirens came and took my father away for the night.

We weren't allowed to talk about what was happening behind closed doors to the outside world, even though the neighbours heard the screams of terror and the thumps of abuse. My father was well-known to the police, and they should have locked him away and buried the key. Sadly, it was a sign of the times when it came to domestic abuse. It was the early 1970s, and back then what happened between husband and wife, stayed behind those tightly closed doors. There was no escape.

I can't even begin to imagine what it was like from my mother's point of view. She married early, a week before she turned 18, and was faced with a violent partner. She was the youngest of three children, with two older brothers, and a dad that idolised her. Sadly, he passed away when I was two, and I don't remember him.

So, picture this. A young woman in her early twenties in the 1970s, with a five-year old and a baby, her own mother grieving the loss of her husband, and she herself, grieving the loss of her father. What a terrible situation that she would have found herself in, with no escape to speak of. She told me once when I asked her why she didn't leave after the first beating; she told me she had been warned that reporting the violence could put her children at risk of removal. Whether that warning was accurate or not, it left her terrified to speak out. She was caught in a web of drunken violence, with no support to speak of.

It wasn't just the violence; it was the quiet afterwards, the pretending that nothing had happened. It was rank with the odour of disgust.

Brief note: Early exposure to violence and neglect can bias a child's stress response toward chronic hyper-activation, particularly in the absence of later corrective experiences. This is where complex trauma can result - not a single event, but the atmosphere of chronic unpredictability. When the body lives too long in that state, it starts mistaking tension for safety, because that's the pattern that's known. It becomes the norm. That confusion can echo later in friendships, work, and intimacy. Ignoring stress doesn't make it vanish; over time, it may shape how comfort and regulation are sought. Many children in these environments learn to earn safety rather than experience it consistently from a parent. A child learns to earn safety instead of it coming naturally from a parent.

My father's volatility and violence grew. When he drank, he punched doors, walls, and my mother. After the standard drunken rage, the following few days he would fill in the holes of the punched doors with putty, and it was never spoken about. He was simply erasing evidence of the violence in his mind. The thing was, he never painted over the putty. So, every time I walked past a door in any one of our houses we lived at, the big grey patches in the middle of the doors were a reminder of his violence.

I suppose the putty for the doors and the gifts to my mum was meant to make his violence easier to erase, and I would have to pretend happy families and forget everything I'd seen, heard, and felt. I desperately wanted a happy family, and instead, I lived my life in constant terror at home. It was abysmal.

On the odd occasion my father came home happy, and those times were great. If he was in the door by 5:45pm during the week, it was a good day. I at least knew mum wasn't going to get beaten, and he might be in a good mood. However, there was a window between 5:45 and 6:30pm which was the 'watch and wait', in case he'd been caught in traffic or held up at work. After 6:30pm, if there was no sign of him, it was danger Will Robinson. I knew what was coming.

We moved again after the landlords who lived behind us had had enough. This time, it was to an apartment in another suburb, which meant I had to change schools. I liked my new school, and teacher, and made new friends, which was comforting. We learnt cursive writing, sewing, and learnt to play sport. At home it was very different. It was learning to quietly survive.

At the time, no one shone a light on domestic violence. Everyone kept to themselves; it was between husband and wife. One time though, his rage was witnessed by everyone at a barbecue held by their fleeting friends. Myself, and everyone else in the backyard, witnessed my father dragging mum by the hair along the ground in front of the barbecue, where other men were cooking sausages. They restrained him, which resulted in the police being called. I gathered the other children there inside to watch TV, to drown out the noise. It was mortifying for everyone who saw the explosion of violence from him. The police took him away for the night, again.

The cycle repeated itself. The police, the following day's silence, the day after having to act like nothing happened. It was the treadmill of terror.

Sometimes mum drove us around late at night, searching pubs and club carparks for his car, so she could work out how to keep us safe for the night. Other times she hid her and us under beds or in wardrobes. Everything she did was driven by fear and survival. I learned to breathe shallowly, so he wouldn't hear me when he came home. He would rage around the house, and we stayed deathly still until we could hear him snoring. Sometimes she would use the food money in desperation to book a motel room for us, or we would sleep in the car. Whatever she could do because it kept escalating.

At that house my father tried to end his life twice, razor blades down his arms once, and with pills another time. The neighbours called the ambulance the second time, and he was taken away to spend some time in an institution.

I do believe we lived close to poverty, though it might not have looked like it from the outside. I remember at that time I had three pairs of underwear, a few second-hand clothes items, two treasured pairs of shoes, and a brown striped dress my gran had bought me at Christmas.

In my head, I had to look after mum. I learnt how to iron the clothes, so she didn't have to. I made her cups of tea. I didn't ask for anything.

Through it all, I clung to school. At primary school I had quite a few friends. Mr Hamill, my teacher in Year 5 believed in me. He was kind, and through his actions, I got to go on a school excursion for free. I sang off-key in the school choir and loved the musicals where I could dance. I even remember the musicals we performed, Pocahontas, and Joseph and his Amazing Technicolour Dream Coat. I practised every day and loved the dancing in them; it was so freeing. I joined the softball team and was even made Sports House Captain the following year.

Dad returned home again after the institution. I think it was only for a week or two before it was rinse and repeat with the drunken violence. Home remained silent the mornings after his benders. Mum wouldn't speak to him, so he addressed us directly; we had no choice, we had to answer and pretend everything was good. Sometimes mum would get new clothes or a different car as another silent, fucked up apology.

The only truly safe place was gran's house - unless dad arrived pounding on her door.

This was my education: how to read the room fast, how to sense when danger was coming, how to disappear. Yet, it was also where my adaptability, observation, and discipline were born. I learnt to read unspoken shifts in the moods of other people. The silent communication from a hypervigilant nervous system. Always on alert, always looking to see where the closest escape route was, always wanting my mum to be safe. I was also becoming increasingly parentified by checking my mum's needs all the time.

Chronic childhood trauma isn't always a single incident; it can be due to the environment that the child is living in. The child's brain learns to manage threat rather than explore life. Hypervigilance becomes a skill for survival. Dissociation feels like calm. Achievement becomes the only safe way to exist.

The body runs on sustained cortisol and adrenaline. Yet, those same neurochemical states sharpen perception and focus, in a constant state of fight or flight. Neglect teaches invisibility; violence teaches anticipation. Every coping strategy can be dialled down over time with the right recognition and management.

# Reflections

Early environments shape the nervous system in ways that are repeatedly shown across trauma science, attachment theory and neurobiology. The body responds to what's happening around it long before someone has the language to make sense of the situation. These aren't personality traits developing, they're physiological adaptations to a world that feels unpredictable (Gunnar & Quevedo, 2007; Schore, 2001).

The amygdala, which is located in the brain, governs the instinctive response to threat we have as humans (it's sometimes referred to as the reptilian brain). It can temporarily override reflective processing, particularly under perceived threat because its prime motivation is to keep you safe by detecting danger. Rational thought and clear decision- making take a back seat when the amygdala is accessing what's called implicit memory. It's the unconscious, long-term memory that affects our behaviour without intention; it's automatic.

Emotional regulation comes more from the prefrontal cortex in the brain, which is associated with executive decision-making, planning, strategy, problem solving and working memory recall. This is quietened when there is the thought of a direct threat to stay safe. This is one of the reasons why there can be confusion and brain fog, when someone has been under long-term stress.

One of the strongest themes in the literature is that chronic stress during childhood activates the stress response system in a long term, cumulative way. The nervous system becomes increasingly oriented toward threat detection, anticipating danger, and keeping the body braced for what comes next. The scientific term for this is allostatic load, and it refers to the wear and tear that builds up when the system is activated too often, with too little recovery time (McEwen & Stellar, 1993; McEwen, 2007).

Attachment research also explains a lot about how children adapt. When care is inconsistent, distracted, frightening, or emotionally unavailable, the child's system learns to navigate the relationship with strategies that maximise safety including staying quiet, becoming hyperaware, pleasing, overperforming, or withdrawing. These strategies are adaptive responses, not signs of deficiency (Bowlby, 1988).

Exposure to ongoing conflict or household instability has its own documented impact. Children who grow up around volatility often become finely tuned to micro-shifts in tone, expression, or body language, because the brain learns that these shifts predict what will happen next (Perry & Szalavitz, 2017). What is often labelled as hypervigilance is, in context, a logical survival strategy.

Emotional neglect is also well documented in the research. When a caregiver is physically present, but emotionally disengaged, the child's nervous system does not consistently receive co-regulation, instead it's the shared emotional presence that teaches the body how to settle (Porges, 2011). Without that, the child develops independent strategies to manage distress, which can carry forward into adulthood.

Family systems research introduces another layer: parentification. When a child is required to take on responsibilities or emotional roles beyond what is developmentally appropriate, the nervous system adapts by becoming highly responsible, overly vigilant, or focused on maintaining order (Cicchetti & Toth, 2016). These patterns are understandable in context.

Identity formation is also shaped by the environment. Developmental psychology shows that children who receive inconsistent validation, shaming messages, or comparisons may form internal narratives around invisibility, unworthiness, or needing to prove themselves (Schore, 2001). These aren't innate beliefs – they can come from lived experience.

These findings from trauma literature remind us that the body makes sense of the world long before the mind can. The patterns that show up later are not random, nor evidence of failure. They are evidence of a system doing everything it could to manage what was in front of it.

# CHAPTER TWO

## Learning to Hide in Plain Sight

The responses described in this chapter reflect physiological adaptation, not personality traits.

We moved again. This time to a house with three bedrooms, so my sister and I had one each, but it was further away from my school. It was my last year of primary school, and with the new house, came new news. My mother and father sat my sister and I down on the couch and told us she was pregnant. I became a big sister to a little baby boy, just before I started high school.

Now, there was a new dynamic in the family, and I remember at first it was really happy one, with a bouncing baby boy. That Christmas, before starting at my new school, my gran bought me a leather briefcase with my initials embossed on it, and a school blazer for my new school. I loved them. I was worried about high school because of the house move; I was the only student attending from my old primary school, so was losing my school friends, in the hope of making new ones.

I arrived at high school expecting to do well. I'd loved primary school - it had been my sanctuary- and my grades had earned me a place in the top class. But the first couple of years at my new school were devastating and devaluing.

As I mentioned, I was the only person that had come across from my primary school. At the orientation, I saw three girls from my preschool, yet none of them were in my class. The loneliness was immediate, and at recess and lunch time I sat alone. The other girls in my class decided that I would be a fabulous target for bullying, and they were merciless. Even my geography teacher smirked while they taunted me. My first report card from her, placed me last in the class with a note that I, "was in the wrong class." I went from a confident over-achiever at school, to the quiet mouse who spoke only when called on. Even then I would hesitate, because whatever I said was mocked or demeaned.

In that first year, the school decided to have a non-uniform day. I hadn't heard the announcement because I'd been home sick. A kind girl in my class found my number in the phone book and told me, though also warned me not to tell anyone she'd let me know about the day (shout out to Sharon). I spent the night terrified it was a trick. That's how confused and brittle I'd become.

By the second year at school, the bullying had eroded my will to attend any classes. I withdrew for three months, too anxious to leave the house. When my mother finally spoke to the school, the year master, Mrs Osborne, paired me with the senior prefects and they became a buffer of safety.

Outside of school, CB radios connected me to new friends. My father had bought them, and we were allowed to talk on them with his control. Through them, I discovered water-skiing and weekends at the beach. This provided me with an escape, both from some of the school issues and what was happening at home.

That same year, a science teacher, who also choreographed the school musicals, noticed I could dance during the musical auditions and I gained a place as one of the dancers. She also forced one of the bullies to lend me her science notebook, so I could copy missed work. I worked really hard to get my grades back to where they should be. The bullying had really taken a toll, and having a science teacher that believed I could do it, made all the difference.

The science teacher cast me front and centre during the dance routines in 'Oklahoma!' in the second year of school, and 'The Boyfriend' in the third year. I loved performing dance routines and it gave me great joy and the camaraderie that I'd been craving.

By Year 9, I'd slipped from the top class in mathematics, to the third lowest. Determined, I had fought my way back up to the middle class by the following year.

Slowly, I rebuilt competence and confidence at school. I joined a group of people who played handball at lunch. This introduced me to a group of girls in my year, and new bonds were formed.

Unfortunately, though, family life and house deteriorated, as my school life slowly improved. Black mould was growing all over my bedroom wall and there was constant moisture dripping down, feeding it. The source of the mould was never investigated, and it wasn't cleaned off until I discovered a mould remover at the supermarket I worked at. Looking back, I suspect it was broken roof tiles; but given it was a rental, I'm not sure that the landlord would have fixed it back then anyway.

There were many pets; dogs, ducks, chickens, rabbits, tortoises rotated through the household, which I look back at with fondness and sadness; it gave me a love of animals, though they were not always well looked after.

My father's volatility continued. If I rose early to shower before school, he would turn on the cold tap in the kitchen, so scalding water blasted from the showerhead, burning me regularly. I once arrived at the school bus stop with shampoo still in my hair, sobbing. A girl on the bus told the school counsellor when we got to school, who called me in to chat. I was mortified and frightened. I refused to speak to him, because weren't allowed to talk about what was happening at home. His solution was to put a blank writing pad in front of me with a pen.

For the first couple of sessions, I wrote nothing, then by about the third or fourth session, I started writing and everything poured out onto the paper. He became my counsellor until I finished school, and four decades later, we're still connected on social media. I can thank him for starting my writing journey.

My mother had another baby, and before the year was over, I had a second baby brother. Two older girls, two baby boys. A chaotic house full of kids, animals, and volatility.

By the following year and with the addition of a fourth child, my parents together discussed that I should leave school and my father organised for me to work with a relative. I begged them to stay in school, because I bloody well needed an education. My father's response? He forbade homework, forcing me to sit on the couch instead of doing it. By then, I was almost fifteen and was working at a supermarket and could buy my own textbooks and school lunches, so that was sorted. I asked my gran if I could move in with her, and she said yes. For the first time in my life, I had a freshly pressed, clean uniform that I didn't have to iron myself, and breakfast waiting. It felt like stepping into a completely different life. Her patience with me as a teenager was amazing, and I have lifelong gratitude for her. I miss my grandmother so much since her passing.

At school I began to flourish because I finally had a social group, and I was elected prefect. The prefect master even sent my parents a congratulatory card, and I was hoping they would be proud. But they never came to the welcome ceremony. I guess I was used to no-shows and disappointments, though this one was unexpected, and hurt. I very much doubt my father would have let my mother attend.

As a clinician now, I look back and feel tenderness for the girl I was.

The constant fight-or-flight. The emotional neglect. The physical neglect. The mould exposure. The humiliation. The nervous-system dysregulation. The people-pleasing. The shame. The fawning. The lack of safety anywhere, except at my gran's place.

If that girl walked into my clinic today, I would immediately support her immune function.

Calm her nervous system. Replenish her depleted micronutrients. Treat her chronic inflammation. Help her regulate her sleep. She was already seeing the school counsellor, so he would be able to determine her level of danger. If she wasn't, I would refer her on to a therapist for help. Duty of care would have to ensure she was in a safe environment.

# Reflections

Adolescence is a period where the brain is wiring itself for identity, belonging, and independence, and research shows that earlier stress patterns don't just disappear when someone reaches high school. They tend to intensify under pressure. The nervous system brings every previous lesson forward into the new environment, especially when safety or acceptance feels uncertain (Schore, 2001; Gunnar & Quevedo, 2007).

Social stress during adolescence is one of the most thoroughly studied areas in developmental psychology. The peer group becomes a central source of belonging, and when bullying or exclusion occurs, the nervous system responds with the same circuitry activated by other forms of interpersonal threat. This activation can influence concentration, digestion, sleep, immunity and mood regulation (Cicchetti & Toth, 2016; McEwen, 2007). These are physiological reactions, not character statements.

Being placed in a new environment, without social support, also appears repeatedly in the literature. When an adolescent enters a group where alliances are already established, the brain leans heavily on earlier-developed survival strategies- staying alert, withdrawing, reading micro-signals, suppressing expression, or finding pockets of safety wherever they appear (Perry & Szalavitz, 2017). These patterns form because the system is doing its best to stay regulated.

Inconsistent belonging - one group offering acceptance while another rejects - creates another predictable pattern. Trauma and attachment research shows that when acceptance fluctuates, the nervous system becomes even more sensitive to social cues, because belonging feels conditional (Bowlby, 1988; Porges, 2011). This creates a survival strategy centred on anticipating others' needs and responses.

Emotional invalidation during adolescence also has a clear footprint in the literature. When teachers, caregivers, or peers minimise or dismiss emotional experiences, the adolescent brain can form internal narratives around being "too much," "oversensitive," or fundamentally wrong in their reactions (Linehan, 1993; Schore, 2001). These beliefs don't develop in a vacuum - they develop through repeated relational and environmental cues.

Adolescents who take on adult responsibilities -whether through work, caring for others, or managing household instability - often develop patterns of functional hyper-independence. The research describes this as a stress adaptation, where the body chooses self-reliance, because co-regulation isn't consistently available (Cicchetti & Toth, 2016). Again, this isn't a personality trait. It's a nervous system strategy.

Physical symptoms during this time are also documented across PNI (psychoneuroimmunology) and stress physiology literature. Chronic stress during adolescence can impact immune function, pain sensitivity, and vulnerability to infections (McEwen & Stellar, 1993; Porges, 2011). These patterns reflect the load on the system, not personal failure.

The evidence across all these fields points to one clear message: adolescent responses make sense when viewed through the lens of what came before. The system doesn't forget. It adapts. And those adaptations are often the very reason a young person gets through those years at all.

# CHAPTER THREE

# Relationship Dynamics

I've had my fair share of encounters with narcissistic traits within intimate relationships. There are experiences I am not able to personally share for various reasons. What I can say is this: I have lived through terrible and deeply cruel dynamics, and that lived experience is what gives me a grounded understanding of how these patterns unfold in real life - not just in theory.

What follows in the next chapter are not individual case studies of specific people. They are conglomerates - composites put together from the many stories I have witnessed and held space for over the years. They reflect recurring patterns, not singular identities. Any resemblance to anyone living or deceased is purely coincidental.

These examples are offered to illuminate what can occur inside relationships where narcissistic traits or behaviours are present- the slow erosion, the confusion, the control dynamics, the toll on the body, and the lasting imprint these experiences can leave behind.

This chapter is about recognising that toxic traits can come in many subtle and different forms.

All cases in this chapter as mentioned before are composite, de-identified clinical portraits drawn from recurring therapeutic patterns observed across many individuals. They do not represent any single real person.

## Angela - Choosing Stability that Looked Like Safety

Angela built a life that others described as calm. Evenings followed a rhythm that rarely changed. Dinner was expected to be on the table by the six o'clock news. The television would be switched on to the same channel every night. It would happen without discussion. It wasn't demanded overtly. It was simply *how things were done.*

In the early years, she interpreted this as structure. Reliability. Normality. After an upbringing shaped by emotional volatility, her routine felt soothing. It gave her nervous system something predictable to anchor to.

Angela and her partner almost never went out for meals.

When friends suggested restaurants or casual dinners, his response was simple: *"Why would we go out? You can cook."*

Angela took this as a compliment. She prided herself on her food. On providing. On being capable. It felt like appreciation, rather than restriction. And because it was framed as admiration, she didn't recognise it as limitation at all.

This is how control often enters - **through quiet manipulation disguised as validation.**

Her body initially experienced these routines as fine and part of domestic life. The scanning that had once kept her hyper-alert eased slightly. To a system shaped by early inconsistency, predictability feels like safety.

But slowly, something else began to appear.

She noticed she rarely chose when or what they ate anymore, only how to execute what was expected. If she suggested eating out, the idea dissolved quickly and without debate. If dinner ran late, the atmosphere changed - not with overt anger, but with pressure she could feel in the room before a word was even spoken.

She began timing her body to the clock.

In quieter moments, she noticed herself delaying hunger until it was "appropriate" to eat. Eating any earlier felt wrong. She would 'sneak' a snack, if she had hidden one in her bedroom drawer. Her husband would eat treats all the time, telling her that 'if you snooze you lose', but would never offer or save any for her. She began suffering from hypoglycaemia. The routine no longer supported her, it **organised her**.

At social gatherings, she stood half a step behind him without noticing she had moved there. In conversations, she softened statements before speaking. She filtered opinions automatically. None of this was driven by fear of punishment. It was driven by **anticipation of disruption**.

She once paused and said, "I don't feel unsafe. I just don't feel like I'm able to do anything outside of the set routine." She wanted some help with her hypoglycaemia symptoms, along with what she had already discussed with her doctor.

This account illustrates patterns described in trauma and attachment literature, where predictability exists without mutual responsiveness. The sympathetic alarm may quiet because overt danger is absent. But true parasympathetic settling never fully arrives, because the relational environment is not mutually responsive.

Her energy was being affected. Laughter became quieter. She would experience trembling. Fatigue appeared that sleep did not resolve. She experienced anxiety and difficulty concentrating.

The internal reference point-the sense of what *she* wanted-grew faint.

The insight came one evening while she was chopping vegetables at the bench, racing against the clock, before it was six o'clock, as she had done thousands of times before. Without drama, without panic, she realised:

She knew exactly when dinner was meant to be ready. She could not remember the last time they had gone out to a restaurant or had eaten a take-away meal.

What she had mistaken for safety, was in fact **the reliable absence of disruption**, not the felt presence of shared decision-making.

And her body had been registering that truth for years - with her symptoms of flatness, quiet fatigue, and the gradual retreat from spontaneous joy.

## Rachael - When "Practical" Quietly Became Conditional

Rachael described her life as "efficient." Everything had a place. Bills were paid on time. Plans were structured. From the outside, it looked organised and calm. There were no dramatic confrontations that neighbours could overhear. No public scenes, and no visible chaos.

And yet, she arrived to the clinic exhausted, in a way that sleep could not repair.

At first, her symptoms dominated our conversations: jaw tension so severe she cracked a molar, shallow breathing that made her sigh constantly without noticing she was doing it, and ongoing upper back pain. She laughed when she spoke about stress, as if it were a personality trait, rather than a physiological state.

The relational pattern emerged slowly.

Money had become centrally controlled over time. At first, it had been presented as practical-one account, one manager, fewer moving parts. That sounded like relief. But eventually, she no longer had independent access to finances at all. If she needed money, she had to **ask her partner for it**.

Not negotiate.
Not plan together.
Ask.

At first, she told herself it was temporary. Then she told herself it didn't matter. Then she stopped noticing how deeply it mattered after all.

She began mentally rehearsing requests before speaking. Groceries. Petrol. Replacing worn shoes. Each need passed through an invisible internal gatekeeper:

*Is this worth asking for? Is this going to become uncomfortable? Will I be questioned?*

One afternoon she was with some friends in a shopping centre, holding a sarong she liked. It was nothing extravagant. Soft. Pastel colours. Something she rarely allowed herself. Her chest tightened. Her breath shortened. She put it back on the rack, without fully understanding why. Her friends asked why she didn't buy it. She told them, "It's sixteen dollars, it's too much". Her friends raised their eyebrows but said nothing. Later that night, she realised: she was unable to even spend sixteen dollars without permission. She also realised that she had to ask for five dollars for her and the children, in case she wanted to buy them an ice cream or grab a loaf of bread, when they were out for a walk or at the park. But, she was told no; it was a waste of money. Her partner went shopping with her for the groceries, and he advised what could and couldn't be bought for the weekly shop. Her husband, though, had no issue going overseas on "mate's trips", or going out for meals with mates where he sprung for the meal.

Clothing became another quiet battleground.

She would get dressed to go out, step into the hallway, and be stopped- not with shouting, not with overt commands, but with questioning.
*"You're wearing that?"*
*"Don't you think that's a bit much?"*
*"People will think the wrong thing."*
*"You should change."*

And she did.

Over time, she learned to pre-empt the commentary, by editing herself before it ever arrived. Higher neckline. Longer hem. Less colour. Fewer decisions that might attract notice. Eventually, she lost touch with what she actually liked to wear at all.

Her body tracked the cost precisely.

Persistent sympathetic activation. Tight back and shoulder muscles. Teeth clenching, particularly in sleep. The nervous system had learned that **visibility carried consequence**.

From a trauma physiology perspective, this creates a very specific internal configuration: the system associates self-expression with risk. So, it chooses concealment as safety. Not because someone is weak, but because withdrawal has become protective.

What destabilised Rachael the most was not deprivation; it was **conditional existence**.

Everything required approval.

Control does not always announce itself with force.

Often it arrives through **the slow disappearance of unedited selfhood.**

## Nicole - When the Body Ends the Conversation

Nicole didn't come to clinic to talk about her relationship. She came because she was anxious and had palpitations that she'd already had medically assessed.

Her first episode happened in a supermarket. No warning. Her heart rate spiked and she felt like she was running a marathon. She felt dizzy and nauseous. Luckily, she was with a friend, who held onto her, so she didn't fall, and instructed her to breathe until it passed.

After that, the episodes kept coming.

She went through every medical test they could think of. ECGs. Blood tests. Monitoring. Everything came back "normal." There was nothing structurally wrong with her heart. However, that didn't match what she was experiencing in her body.

The night that changed things was having to go to hospital because her heart rate would not decrease.

She was lying in the bed, with monitors attached, while her heart rate stayed high without any clear reason. Staff were coming and going. It was clinical and busy. What stayed with her wasn't the machines or the doctors - it was how alone she felt while her body was in distress, even though her partner was there. When he was told by the doctor that she may have had a heart attack, he replied, "Oh yeah?" and went back to the newspaper he had brought with him to read. The doctor said to him, "You realise this is very serious? "He shrugged, and kept on reading, almost dismissing the doctor's presence. No emotion.

Later she said, "My body thought I might die, and at the same time it felt like no one was really there with me."

After that, her system stopped settling.

Panic started showing up in everyday places. In the car. At home. At work. Sleep became broken. Her appetite dropped off. Sudden noises made her jump. Her body was permanently on alert. Her partner wasn't home much, he was always busy at the gym, or out with his friends, or had work events to attend outside of business hours.

What confused her was that nothing "big" had happened that she could point to. No single incident that explained the level of fear in her nervous system. Until she found out from one of his colleagues that her partner had been cheating on her with someone from the office. She said later that "I knew something was off, but couldn't put my finger on it, and any questions initially were met with, "you're being paranoid again," "don't be so dramatic," and "I work so hard for us, you should be more grateful."

One day she said, "It feels like my body left before I did." Her nervous system had drawn a boundary before her conscious mind was ready to.

But that's how the body works under long-term relational strain. The amygdala doesn't wait for one dramatic event. It learns from repeated stress and unpredictability. And once it decides the environment isn't safe, it acts without consulting the thinking brain.

## Poppy - Pregnancy, Vulnerability and Emotional Absence

Poppy went into pregnancy believing it would stabilise everything. She thought becoming a family would naturally bring more closeness and support.

Her physical recovery was hard. Blood loss due to anaemia. She had an infection that saw her readmitted to hospital, and she needed a round of IV antibiotics. From there, she had ongoing exhaustion with a new baby and was trying her best to recover after the birth. Her sleep was broken, and her body needed far more support than she had ever needed before.

And in that vulnerability, something registered.

There was no yelling.
No obvious abandonment.
No dramatic cruelty.

There was simply no one there for her in the way she needed. Her husband and mother-in-law criticised how she did things as a standard way of life for her, and her mother and father were just never there for her.

She told me about sitting on the edge of the bed one night feeding the baby. And the thought that landed was very clear.

"I am doing this on my own, I need help, not criticism."

After the birth, the stock standard reassurance that everyone says:

"It'll get better, and you'll forget all about this when the baby is older."
"You'll be fine."
"This is just the hard part," no longer meant anything.

None of it settled her system anymore. It wasn't getting better, because although she had the picture-perfect life from the outside, she had no internal support, empathy, help, or validation.

She didn't leave straight away. She stayed for many years, so lonely in her marriage, except for her child. Eventually, her husband told her that he had never wanted children (though that was one of the values that initially drew her to him, as he'd told her he did), and he didn't like being second to a child. She noted that her husband said second and she queried him on it. He said the child was now her priority, he was second and she was last.

What changed first was her expectation. She stopped assuming emotional availability, where it hadn't actually been present.

That was the point where she began to see the relationship clearly, instead of hopefully. They divorced, she met a man with a big extended family who valued her and her child, and he was happy to become a stepfather. She had a child with her second partner, and had a completely different pregnancy, birth, and post-partum experience. It was one of joy instead of loneliness.

## Eloise - Illness without Support

Eloise's health declined over a few years, not suddenly, incrementally. Repeated infections. Exhaustion that never really lifted, akin to chronic fatigue. She kept functioning because that's what she had always done, but she was adrenally exhausted.

What made it harder was that she wasn't believed.

When she said she was exhausted, she was told she was overreacting.
When she said she didn't feel well, she was told it was anxiety. When she said something felt wrong in her body, she was told it was "all in her head."

After a while, she stopped saying it out loud.

She still went to appointments. Still took medication. Still managed symptoms quietly. But inside the relationship, her fatigue and illness were treated as exaggeration, rather than reality.

That does something very specific to a person.

Her body was struggling, and at the same time she was being told her experience wasn't real. So she started questioning herself instead of the situation. She pushed harder. Rested less. Explained more. Apologised for being unwell.

Her body stayed permanently tight. She said she felt so exhausted that even getting up in the morning felt like walking through waist-deep mud.

During one visit she said, very simply, "I think I've been alone in this relationship for a long time."

There was no anger in it. Just clarity.

That was the moment the self-blame started to loosen. She had spent years believing she wasn't coping properly. Once she named the reality of being unwell and not believed, her symptoms stopped feeling like personal failure and started making sense as a response to long-term strain.

Her body hadn't been weak.

It had been carrying illness and disbelief at the same time.

## Jennifer - The Exit Begins in the Body

Jennifer didn't plan to leave her marriage; her belief was that she made a vow when she got married and that was her lot in life. It was her body that started withdrawing, before her mind caught up.

Sex with her husband became something she avoided. When it did happen, she felt sick afterwards, and she often vomited at work the next day. Her colleagues covered for her, without needing explanations, because she often showed up for work or work events in tears because he'd started an argument with her just before she was due to be somewhere. She advised that her husband called her names like "loser" instead of Jennifer and repeatedly told her she was "damaged goods" because she'd had children, so no-one else would want her. He was financially controlling, and he constantly demeaned her privately and after a while, publicly. He told her that if he wanted to end the marriage, he would make it unbearable for her, so that she'd have to leave and he wouldn't look like the bad guy to their friends and family. Her nervous system had already drawn a line she hadn't yet felt brave enough to draw herself.

When she finally got to breaking point and told her husband it was over, he agreed very quickly and moved onto a woman he'd been working with.

They had to stay living under the same roof after the separation, until the house was sold. Her body stayed in constant alert, because he became more and more volatile to try and force her to move out. It was unbearable at times for her and she was very lucky to have support from good friends who helped her through it.

She still showed up for work. Still got the children to school. Still managed day-to-day life. But inside, her system never stood down.

She later said that the relationship itself had been hard, but ending it nearly broke her.

That makes sense physiologically. When there's no stable bond and no clean separation, the body stays trapped in threat response.

Jennifer didn't leave because she felt strong.

She left because her body stopped allowing her to stay.

## Letisha -Aftermath – When a Relationship is Over, is it Really?

Letisha came to clinic many years after her relationship had ended, with digestive issues that were labelled as irritable bowel syndrome. She had had this syndrome for fifteen years, and she recalled it had begun around the same time that she was waiting for her divorce to come through.

Her body had been on edge because the situation stayed unstable. What affected her most were ongoing disruptions involving the children. Pick-ups that changed without warning. School arrangements that shifted suddenly. Information delivered late or not at all. Each change pulled her straight back into alert mode.

Plans changed without notice, and she would have to adjust her work and plans accordingly. Information was withheld when the children were ill. Once her husband took her daughters out of school and interstate without telling her, which terrified her. She had no idea where they were.

This is one of the most important realities when you are dealing with someone with **narcissistic traits**:

The relationship may end.
The control often does not.

As long as there are shared children, the dynamic continues through logistics, access, unpredictability, and power. The body never gets clean separation. It stays responsive because it has to.

Letisha told me that even on quiet nights, her digestion would not behave. Nothing was happening in that moment -but she was trying to work out if stress made it far worse, or if it was the irritable bowel stressing her more.

She still worried about her children's whereabouts, even though they were now adults. Her nervous system didn't stay activated because she "couldn't move on." It stayed activated because she had lived with a very unpredictable situation for over fifteen years.

For Letisha, real settling didn't begin until we worked on settling the symptoms of irritable bowel down and then started working on nourishing her nervous system with supplements and herbal medicine.

## Claire- Aftermath, When a Pet Becomes a Pawn

Claire came to clinic after the relationship had ended. On paper, it was over. They were no longer living together. The separation had happened.

But the behaviour hadn't stopped.

When Claire left, her and the children had to move in with friends for a while. It wasn't permanent, just somewhere to land until she could find a place of her own. Because of that, she couldn't take Citrine with her straight away.

Citrine was her ragdoll cat. The constant through everything.

The agreement was that once Claire found a place of her own, she would come back and get Citrine. That was always the plan.

When she finally moved into a house, she contacted her ex and told him she was ready to bring Citrine home. He agreed without hesitation and arranged for her to collect her on a day when he would be home. It was close to Christmas. She felt relieved knowing she'd have Citrine back with her and the kids.

Something didn't quite sit right though.

So, just in case, she went to the rescue shelter and brought home a new kitten. She told herself having two cats would be fine, and Citrine would adjust. She rang her husband ahead of time to ensure she was home so she could collect Citrine.

That's when he told her he had given Citrine away.

Not to a stranger.
Not to a shelter.

To his niece, who didn't get along with Claire.

No discussion.
No warning.
No chance to say goodbye.

That moment was a breaking point for her.

She didn't show it. She still got up the next day. Still took the kids where they needed to go. Still answered messages. Still kept herself together on the outside. If you looked at her life, you wouldn't have suspected anything had cracked.

But inside, something finally gave way.

It didn't affect the children because there was a new kitten at home. Thank goodness she hadn't told them that Citrine was coming back.

But for Claire, the meaning was unmistakable.

When it's over, the relationship may end.
But when you're dealing with someone with narcissistic traits, the need to control often doesn't.

The animal wasn't the point.
The power was.

Claire kept functioning. Kept managing the children. Kept rebuilding the practical side of life. After that though, she repeatedly began getting sore throats and colds, going from one cough or cold every few years, to repeated respiratory tract and throat infections. As soon as she'd recover from one, she'd pick up something new.

She was also suffering from insomnia. It began because she'd lay awake at night wondering how Citrine was and whether she was being looked after properly, and it had become a habit where she'd wake numerous times each night. To counteract this, we worked on strengthening her immune and nervous system, and helping her improve her sleep, so she could get some rest and begin the healing journey.

# Reflections

*Body, Survival Physiology, and Coercive Dynamics*

What stands out most across the experiences in this chapter is how consistently the body responds, long before the mind fully understands what is happening.

In every story - Angela, Rachael, Nicole, Poppy, Eloise, Jennifer, Letisha and Claire - the nervous system spoke first. Not in words. Not in decisions. But in fatigue, nausea, racing heart, shallow breath, muscle tension, digestive issues, insomnia, vigilance, shutdown.

Physiologically, threat-detection systems respond to cumulative pattern recognition rather than conscious certainty. In other words, it doesn't require proof. It responds to patterns.

The nervous system is built to answer one primary question:

**Is this environment predictable and safe, or is it unpredictable and threatening?**

When an environment is shaped by control, emotional withdrawal, humiliation, financial restriction, mixed signals, or chronic unpredictability, the body doesn't interpret this as a "relationship problem." It interprets it as **ongoing threat exposure**.

That is why the women in this chapter did not all leave in the same way, at the same time, or for the same visible reasons. Their bodies were responding to a cumulative load, not a single moment.

From a neurobiological perspective, repeated exposure to unpredictable relational environments sensitises the amygdala -

the brain's threat detection centre. Once sensitised, its alarm threshold drops. This is why people become acutely aware of tone changes, facial expressions, timing shifts, silences and micro-signals. The body learns to scan before the thinking brain has time to evaluate.

The vagus nerve which governs calmness, connection, heart rhythm, digestion, and emotional regulation – reduces its tone under chronic relational stress according to polyvagal and autonomic regulation models. Heart rate variability can reduce, breathing can be affected, digestion becomes more reactive, and sleep may be disrupted. The body stays in preparation mode.

This is **adaptive survival physiology**.

Appeasement, shrinking, self-editing, over-explaining, minimising needs, and doubting perception are not personality flaws. They are survival strategies. They are how the nervous system attempts to keep the environment stable enough to survive.

And when appeasement no longer works, the body escalates:

- Panic
- Collapse
- Illness
- Aversion
- Shutdown.

One of the thoughts people might internalise is this:

"If it were really that bad, I would have left sooner."

From an evolutionary and attachment perspective, the body tends to prioritise continuity and attachment over abrupt change. It will tolerate extraordinary internal strain in an attempt to preserve connection, until the physiological cost becomes greater than the cost of leaving. When that threshold is reached, departure often feels abrupt and "out of character."

In reality, it is simply the end of a very long conversation the nervous system has been having quietly with the rest of the body for years.

As seen with Letisha and Claire, post-separation does not automatically mean post-threat, particularly when someone has strong narcissistic traits. The relationship may end, but the control often relocates into logistics, timing, unpredictability, access to children, silence and disruption. The nervous system does not get a clean edge. It remains alert because it has to.

This is why people are often told they are "not moving on" when, in fact, they are still responding accurately to a system that has not yet become safe.

Clinical and physiological models suggest healing often begins when sufficient safety cues allow threat responses to down-regulate. Those safety cues might look like:

- Predictability
- Reduced contact
- Clear boundaries that are enforced rather than negotiated
- Support that is embodied, not just spoken
- Help with nourishing and healing the body
- Nervous system support
- Environments that no longer require constant self-monitoring.

Only then does recalibration begin.

Not all at once.
Not neatly.
But gradually.

Breath deepens.
Sleep lengthens.
Digestion settles.
The heart slows without effort.
The shoulders drop without instruction.

And it happens not through willpower, but through **safety and support repeated often enough to be believed**.

If you recognise yourself in any of these women, the most important thing to understand is this:

Your body has not been betraying you; it's been protecting you, with the only language it has.

Once that's understood, everything changes.

# CHAPTER FOUR

# Work – The Final Bastion

**Part I**

Just like school and learning, I love work and all its challenges. It is where I can make a difference, create 'til my heart's content, and be me.

As a single parent, I worked hard to provide a safe, stable environment for my children, residing around the same area so they could retain their solid friend base, whilst satisfying my craving to help people with my work, whether it be face to face or anonymously. I was lucky, I had a job that was flexible with school holidays, so I was able to spend more time with my children over this period.

During my career, I had become established in the field of complementary medicine and was known for being able to take a product concept from idea to regulatory approval, with precision. I'd created, rebuilt, and refined product lines for multiple companies, and I was deeply trusted because I understood both the science and the practical application. That reputation naturally led me to a role where I was asked to help stabilise and elevate a brand that needed direction.

At first, everything seemed straightforward-busy, but familiar. I was contributing to and writing articles, reviewing educational content and ensuring regulatory compliance. I was doing the type of work that required a great deal of accuracy, and I was good at it.

It wasn't long before I started working closely with a new work colleague, who had come from a completely different professional background, one that didn't include the regulatory frameworks required in complementary medicine. That meant we were often at odds - my role required accuracy, evidence and adherence to strict guidelines, while theirs leaned more toward dramatic messaging.

The more I tried to explain the regulations, the more resistance I faced. At first, it was irritation. Then it escalated to open hostility. They reacted strongly whenever their work required correction, even when those corrections were necessary to protect the business. And because it was a small team, there was no hiding when these reactions happened.

Nothing appeared to soften their hostile responses; in practice, calm responses were often followed by further escalation. It became an environment where I started anticipating conflict, a response consistent with prolonged exposure to interpersonal unpredictability. This isn't a conscious choice; it reflects conditioned threat anticipation shaped by repeated interpersonal stress when someone else's mood becomes unpredictable.

Things shifted again when they began making claims about guidance they said they had received from regulatory bodies - claims that did not align with how regulatory systems actually operate. Regulatory authorities don't give personal advice; they provide guidelines, and those guidelines don't change at the whim of one conversation. When those claims reached the senior executive, I had no choice but to respond with facts.

Providing factual clarification appeared to coincide with increased tension within the dynamic. When my colleague didn't get the response they wanted, the volatility of their responses began to affect the broader working environment It became uncomfortable, unpredictable, and emotionally draining.

Around this time, I consulted an industry colleague who also happened to be a psychologist. After I described what had been happening, they suggested I investigate how narcissistic behaviour can show up in professional settings. I'd always thought of the term "narcissist" as something thrown around lightly, usually referring to someone who liked taking selfies. I didn't associate it with workplace patterns or interpersonal instability.

That conversation changed my view significantly. It led me down a path of research, discovery, and a deeper understanding.

Suddenly, the behaviours I'd been experiencing had a framework. The patterns made sense. The reactions made sense. The escalation made sense.

And for the first time, I realised that the problem wasn't my communication style, my competence, or my emotional stability, it was the dynamic itself.

Once I understood that, I sought the advice of an industry leader to navigate the dynamic. They met with me several times with valuable feedback that I implemented, but it didn't help. They suggested that leaving the situation was the healthiest option, so I stepped away from the role, and that departure became a turning point. It was the first workplace experience that opened the door to understanding narcissistic behaviours as a structured, recognisable pattern - not a personality quirk, not a conflict, not a misunderstanding, but a pattern.

This wasn't the end of my encounters with these personality structures in the workplace, but it was the beginning of my education regarding those types of traits and it planted the seed for everything that would come next.

## Part II

I've been fortunate to work in environments that were genuinely uplifting, collaborative and professionally satisfying. For the most part, my workplace experiences have been positive, encouraging, and filled with people who were passionate about what they did. But there were a small number of situations where the dynamics were different, where certain patterns appeared that mirrored earlier experiences in my life.

What follows is another example of workplace exposure to narcissistic traits I encountered at a different point in my career. It was separate from the situation described earlier, and it stood out because the behavioural patterns on reflection were so familiar, even though the circumstances were entirely different.

I was developing a range of products, working closely with a team responsible for expanding into new markets. It was a good fit for my skill set; formulations, education, research, regulatory knowledge - and the scope was broad enough to be exciting. I initially worked remotely, and the pace was demanding from the outset, with expectations increasing quickly.

Eventually, the workload grew to the point where I had to be in the office, which was quite a distance away. I moved house, and the new environment was quiet, isolating, and very different from what I was used to. It's amazing what a difference a couple of hours travel time make in determining how often you see family and friends. My children were older and wanted to stay put, so our two dogs came with me, and later two cats joined my household. Their presence gave me comfort, but the solitude was something very new to me.

Inside the workplace, I began to notice familiar patterns. A few individuals responded in ways that didn't make sense - undermining, dismissiveness, or questioning based on personal discomfort, rather than scientific or regulatory accuracy. When spoken to individually, they denied any issues. But in group settings, their interactions shifted into something more coordinated and destabilising.

The tone changed again during a performance discussion with a senior executive. Instead of a constructive conversation, they made a dramatic statement about the business not surviving without my contributions. Rather than feeling like recognition, it landed with a kind of weight I couldn't quite articulate, it was weird.

From that point, the dynamic tightened. I continued delivering high-quality formulations, detailed research, and regulatory pathways, but the environment was becoming more destabilising. This pattern was deeply confusing to me at the time.

During this time, the senior executive's behaviour escalated sharply. One day, they called me into a room, closed the door, and accused me of being a "control freak." When I asked for an example so I could modify my behaviour, none could be offered. The conversation moved in circles - contradictory, unclear, and emotionally charged. At one point, they asked why I didn't "fight" with them anymore. I hadn't realised conflict was expected, and the statement made no sense to me. I didn't have any "fight" left in me, it all seemed so ludicrous and confusing.

Then came the whiteboard incident. They told me I couldn't leave the room until I wrote the word control three times on the whiteboard. I genuinely thought they were joking at first. But they weren't. By the time I complied, tears were streaming down my face. I walked back to my desk, gathered my things, and left the building.

On the drive home, my phone rang. It was them.

Their voice was bright and cheerful; "How are you?" Completely disconnected from what had occurred minutes earlier. The emotional disconnect between what had just happened and the tone of that call was extreme. It really was a "What the fuck?" moment.

There were other incidents too. Team gatherings where volatility was directed at me with others present. A new colleague later told me they had been encouraged to provoke me during a meeting, something they later divulged. In that meeting, they raised their voice at me aggressively, and all I could do was ask them to stop yelling at me. Two other colleagues intervened and suggested we take a break. Immediately afterward, the senior executive who orchestrated this, shifted into casual conversation, taking me for a drive to look at the beach as if nothing out of the ordinary had happened. Again, the emotional disconnect was extreme.

That emotional whiplash, the rapid shift from hostility to charming, was destabilising, producing confusion, hypervigilance, and physiological stress. I continued enduring it as long as I safely could. I consulted a doctor, then a psychologist, who advised that the situation was not sustainable and advised me to leave as soon as possible. I made a structured plan. I packed up, sold my car to cover the moving costs, gathered the animals, hired a van, and returned to my support system.

By the time I got back home, I felt stripped back to my foundations. It wasn't only emotional depletion, my body, mind, and spirit had carried far too much for too long.

Yet in that stripped-back space, something important came into focus: this wasn't merely a difficult workplace. It aligned with relational patterns I had since learned to recognise.

The clarity and recognition weren't comfortable, but marked a turning point in how I approached both my work and my healing.

## Part III

## Work Collaboration: the opposite experience.

In my professional community I'd always thrived in environments where respect, curiosity, and shared purpose were the baseline rather than the exception. After a couple of furfies along the way, I can give you an example of what healthy professional collaboration actually looks like. Not the glossy corporate version people perform, but the real thing - where peers share ideas freely, challenge one another respectfully, and work towards something that's bigger than any one of us.

The project that anchored this period for me - and for many of us working together at the time - was the regulatory submission for theanine to be permitted in listed medicines in Australia. I was asked to spearhead the submission, but it was never a solo effort. This was one of those rare industry moments where expertise from all directions lined up neatly: regulatory minds, research-driven clinicians, formulation specialists, and the people who know how to translate dense data into something a regulator can actually evaluate without losing the will to live.

The science itself was fascinating. Theanine's influence on alpha-wave activity, stress modulation, and cognitive calm had been examined internationally for years, and synthesising all that research into a submission and education piece felt like assembling a puzzle where every piece had to be justified, referenced and articulated, without overstating a thing. There's something very grounding about a process where the rules are clear, the evidence is what it is, and no one is trying to distort anything for ego's sake.

The best part? No one was trying to outdo anyone else. No one was sabotaging the process. No one was rooting for someone to fail. It was a group of professionals doing what they do best;

combining decades of knowledge into something that served the wider industry.

The contrast to less functional workplaces was there, of course, but I didn't need to spell it out. It showed itself in the silence - in what wasn't present. No volatility. No walking on eggshells or unpredictability dressed up as "creativity." Just the usual challenge of complex regulatory work, which is more than enough for any normal day.

We worked steadily and thoughtfully, with a kind of unspoken respect that develops among people who care about doing things properly. When the submission was finally approved, it wasn't a triumph for one person. It was a moment that belonged to all of us - a collective achievement built on shared effort, shared expertise, and a shared sense of responsibility.

There was a personal layer to it, too. Not in a dramatic, life-defining way, but in the sense that working on a compound associated with stress physiology and neural calming, had a faintly poetic irony I wasn't oblivious to. My career had always been in complementary medicine - clinic, formulation, research, education - but the deeper I delved into the science of stress, the more it aligned with everything I understood from lived experience. It didn't feel like a reinvention. It felt like integration.

During this time, I began translating the research into education: writing articles, recording podcasts, presenting webinars, and creating content for both practitioners and the public. Teaching is something that has always grounded me. When you explain physiology in plain language - when you help people understand that stress has a structure, a mechanism, and a pattern - it gives them back a bit of agency. It's the opposite of chaos. It's clarity. I had lectured for a few years previously at a naturopathic college in nutritional and herbal medicine subjects, and anatomy and physiology, so this was great fun.

The most satisfying part of this period wasn't the accomplishment itself. It was the reminder that healthy environments exist and that most people genuinely want to collaborate, contribute, and do meaningful work. It was a quiet reassurance that the corrosive dynamics I'd seen were outliers, not a reflection of my industry as a whole.

Most workplaces are not battlegrounds. Most people are not out to harm you. Most collaboration is exactly what it looks like - people doing their jobs with integrity.

This chapter wasn't about recovering from anything. It was about remembering what steady ground feels like. And that remembering becomes part of the healing in its own quiet way.

## Reflections

When you look at what long-term pressure does to a human system, it's clear that the body responds long before your conscious mind catches up. And truly, your system takes notes, even when you're too busy surviving to notice.

It doesn't matter whether the stress comes from a workplace, a relationship, a family, or a combination of all three. The physiology is the physiology. We're built for short bursts of stress, not the slow drip of situations that require you to stay alert, adaptable, or hyper-responsible for too long.

You see this in the research on allostatic load, the cumulative wear and tear caused by repeated activation of the stress response (McEwen & Wingfield, 2003). Over time, cortisol patterns shift, sleep becomes disrupted, inflammation rises, and clarity becomes cloudiness. It's not dramatic; it's incremental, like the body's quiet bookkeeping.

The nervous system also plays a major role here. When you've been in environments where unpredictability is normal, the amygdala in the brain becomes quicker to detect potential threat - not because you're "sensitive," but because that's literally what it's designed to do under chronic stress (LeDoux, 2015). This is neuroplasticity at work. The system adapts to what it believes is necessary for survival.

Add in what polyvagal theory describes as neuroception - the subconscious detection of safety or danger - and you can see why some environments feel warm and supportive, and others feel destabilising, even when the behaviour looks "calm" on the surface (Porges, 2011). The internal gauge is incredibly accurate.

There's also a cognitive element. When behaviour from others is inconsistent, for example, warm one moment, dismissive the next, saying one thing, and then doing the complete opposite, the mind tries to reconcile the mismatch. That internal tug-of-war is commonly described in organisational psychology as cognitive dissonance (Hinojosa et al., 2017). It's not about weakness; it's about the brain trying to create coherence, where coherence doesn't exist.

And when the external world requires you to keep functioning through all of that, the body simply stores the strain. Not in a mystical way, but in a very real neurobiological way. Immune function can shift in chronic stress states (Segerstrom & Miller, 2004). Pain thresholds can be altered due to sensitisation in the nervous system (Fitzcharles et al., 2021). Digestive changes can show up as irritable bowel syndrome; it's physiology under load.

What's important for you to know is this: You don't have to feel "broken" for these patterns to show up. You don't have to meet any diagnostic criteria. You don't even have to realise the load you've been carrying. Human bodies are beautifully loyal. They track what you go through so that you can keep going.

And with the right inputs - consistent support, proper nourishment, safety, boundaries, and tools that let the system downshift - the same body that kept you alive under duress can learn to soften again. That's the part many people don't hear enough: the system is capable of recalibrating.

None of this is about blame. None of this is about pathology. This is simply the biology of being human in a world that sometimes doesn't make sense.

For anyone reading, your body's signals make sense. They're not exaggerations or weaknesses. They're the natural consequences of being a person with a nervous system that was designed to keep you safe.

And if there's one thing decades of research, clinical experience, and lived experience consistently show, it's this: When you give a human system safety, nourishment, rest and clarity it responds. Every time.

# CHAPTER FIVE

# The Apex Break

There comes a point where the body draws a hard line, whether you consent to it or not. Mine arrived quietly, without ceremony, after a long stretch of trying to hold too many things together at once.

I had begun a new role in a vibrant, fast-paced team, it was the kind of environment that energises you and keeps you sharp. It was engaging, dynamic, and full of possibility. My practice was left to weekends or evening appointments.

After years of primarily working remotely, I was suddenly in the office five days a week, so I moved house to be closer to the workplace, which was great place to live. However, I worried about leaving my dogs and cats at home for that long, after so many years of near-constant presence with them. It was a shift in rhythm, and it undoubtedly significantly contributed to my stress levels.

At the same time, someone I cared about deeply was unravelling. A friend who'd lost family members and was injured, needed somewhere to land. So, I opened my home because that's what you do when someone is lost and you have the capacity, or at least, you *think* you do, to help them.

Then came the phone call about another close friend, a call no one wants to receive. They had attempted to be unalive, and I found out by accident during that call, because that someone had been told to withhold the information from me. That was a true blow, fear, sadness, disbelief, and a quiet disappointment at the secrecy all at once.

Then my physical health really gave way. I'd finally reached my physical tipping point.

I had been developing more and more allergies, and was becoming allergic to my pets, a lot of standard foods, dust and pollens. My tongue would get swollen, so I started restricting my diet as much as possible whilst maintaining the right nutrient balance.

I'd had the flu the year before and had experienced shingles for the first time. A tooth infection spiralled into sepsis. It took two rounds of antibiotics before it had to be extracted. My body, already worn down, was in no state to take another hit. I developed shingles again.

That was before my back pain, the one that had been whispering at me for a little while, became something else entirely. The back pain became so aggressive that I couldn't function.

The MRI showed Tarlov cysts. Many people have them without symptoms. Mine, however, decided to make themselves known. I had alternating pain, then numbness going down my groin and the inside of my leg. I also had terrible pain on the outside of my leg, as well as back pain. One of the cysts ruptured and the pain was beyond anything I could have anticipated. I had the worst lower back pain imaginable – it was awful! I couldn't navigate stairs. Sitting hurt. Standing hurt. Lying down was unbearable. Then came the moment I couldn't get out of bed at all. I was so sleep deprived, exhausted and couldn't think straight.

**Sometimes the body steps in when you won't. This chapter starts at the point where everything gave out at once, forcing a halt and creating the space needed to rebuild with intention, rather than sheer momentum.**

And yet, even then, I tried to keep going. I tried to keep supporting my friend who was living with me. I tried to keep working. I tried to keep functioning.

Until one morning I lay in bed and thought: *This is NOT going to be my life. No. I refuse.*

Something in me finally gave way. The part of me that had carried and carried and carried finally put the load down. Maybe it was the pain. Maybe it was the sleep deprivation, due to the pain. Maybe it was the worry about not being able to go to work. I knew I had to make changes right then and there.

I asked my friend to move out. Not because I didn't care, but because I couldn't carry both of us and survive. I cut contact with anyone toxic or draining; I needed to heal without noise.

I resigned from my role. A role I genuinely liked, with people who genuinely supported me, because my body needed a full stop, not a comma.

Then I began the protocol.
My protocol.
The one I designed from every tool I've ever learned:

Movement
Supplements
Herbal medicine
Nervous system support
Nutrition

Homeopathy
Rest
Discipline
Boundaries
Stillness.

Healing didn't arrive dramatically, it came incrementally. Strength returned one layer at a time. My body began to rebuild, and my mind relaxed. Then came the difficult part; facing the grief of removing toxic and draining people. The grief was real. But so was the relief.

By the time I emerged from this period, I was different. Clearer. Stronger. Calmer. More anchored in my purpose than I had been in decades.

This chapter is where everything that came before converged. A full physical breakdown that became the pivot. The moment where survival gave way to recalibration - deliberate, grounded, and entirely on my terms.

# Reflections

There's something very real about what happens when the body finally puts the brakes on after years of cumulative load. It's not theatrical or symbolic. It's simply physiology reaching its tipping point.

A full physical shutdown - whether triggered by infection, chronic pain, exhaustion, or the weight of multiple stressors hitting at once - is often the moment the system asserts itself in a way that can't be ignored. This isn't weakness; it's the body protecting its own integrity.

In the research on allostatic load, this is described as the point where the stress-response machinery has been activated so many times for so long that the system begins shifting from adaptation to depletion (McEwen & Wingfield, 2003). It's cumulative. Incremental. The kind of thing that builds quietly, until it doesn't.

Pain escalation follows a similar pattern. When the nervous system has been exposed to chronic stress, the threshold for pain can lower, due to sensitisation pathways becoming more reactive (Fitzcharles et al., 2021). The pain isn't imagined and it isn't exaggerated - it's mediated by the interaction between the sensory nerves, the spinal cord, and the brain's threat-monitoring networks.

Layer in what we know from psychoneuroimmunology, and it makes sense that infections can hit harder when the system is under strain. Chronic stress can influence immune efficiency, inflammatory responses, and recovery rate (Segerstrom & Miller, 2004). Again, this isn't about character or resilience. It's biology doing exactly what biology does under pressure.

From a nervous-system perspective, moments like these often represent what polyvagal theory would describe as a "shutdown" response - a move toward immobilisation when the system perceives that continued mobilising is no longer viable (Porges, 2011). It's the body's version of saying: *enough*.

What is important to highlight is that recovery from this kind of collapse is rarely spontaneous. It's iterative, slow, and built from consistent, small adjustments; the kinds of things that support the system in recalibrating, rather than compensating.

Movement in measured doses.
Nourishment that supports physiological repair.
Rest structured in ways the body can actually use.
Boundaries that reduce unnecessary activation.
Herbal, homeopathic, and nutritional support with mechanisms that align with what the system needs.

What the research continually shows is that the human body has enormous capacity for restoration when given the right conditions. Neuroplasticity supports the gradually shifting of pain patterns (Apkarian et al., 2011). Stress-circuitry can recalibrate when the load changes. Immune markers improve when the system exits chronic activation.

Nothing about this is linear. Nothing about it is instant. But it *is* possible - and often surprisingly responsive - once the burden that caused the collapse is removed.

For anyone reading, the takeaway is simple:

A physical shutdown doesn't mean failure.
It doesn't mean fragility.
It means your system has been paying attention.

Bodies are honest. Your body doesn't lie. It tells the truth before the mind is ready to acknowledge it. And when it finally insists on rest, it's not a punishment. It's an invitation to rebuild differently - with clarity, capacity, and better footing than before.

# CHAPTER SIX

# Stabilisation and Insight

Coming out the other side of a collapse is not a cinematic moment. There's no triumphant music, no sudden clarity, no instant wisdom. It's much quieter than that. More deliberate. More practical. Integration isn't a rebirth in the dramatic sense; it's simply the point where things start landing properly in the system again.

The first stage of pulling myself back up wasn't about emotional clarity or newfound boundaries - it was physical. I focused on gradually stabilising my body, because nothing else made sense until that was sorted. Recovery started with the basics: managing the pain, moving when I could, resting when I had to, and getting through the practical tasks in front of me.

My animals were with me through all of it. When I was bedbound, they stayed close in the natural way animals do when they sense you're not yourself. Feeding them, caring for them, keeping their routine going - that became the anchor. It gave me structure, when everything else was stripped back. It kept me connected to something steady, when my own body was unpredictable.

There was nothing profound about this stage. It was survival, discipline, and looking after the creatures who relied on me. That was the real beginning of integration: doing what needed to be done until my system started to trust that the crisis had passed.

As my body stabilised, everything else began to sift into place. My back pain became more intermittent than constant. Energy returned in increments. The constant internal strain that comes from carrying too much for too long began to settle. When the body isn't in crisis, you can finally assess what's actually happening, instead of reacting to every flare, spike, or demand.

Clarity arrived slowly, folded into ordinary moments, rather than revelations. It wasn't about reinvention, it was more about nurturing myself after many years of strain. The practical decisions became easier. What I would accept. What I wouldn't. What aligned. What didn't. Not rigid. Just clear.

My work started to feel cohesive again - not as a distraction, but as something that naturally integrated who I am: the clinician, the researcher, the educator, the woman who understands stress and physiology, not just from textbooks, but also from lived experience. The threads began to align, because my system finally had the capacity to hold them.

I grieved too, but grief wasn't the whole story. It was just one part of integration - the clearing out before the rebuild.

Rebirth, for me, wasn't about becoming someone new. I'm too old for that, and I happen to like who I am. It wasn't a reinvention or a makeover of the self. It was incremental, practical, and grounded. I stopped pouring energy into what drained me.

And slowly, when you take the time to heal from a whole-body point of view, you become someone who functions from steadiness instead of urgency - someone whose body, mind, and boundaries are finally moving in the same direction.

This chapter wasn't about recovery in the inspirational sense. It was about living differently, because there was finally enough internal room to do so.

# Reflections

When you strip everything back and the body finally has room to recalibrate, the science behind it is remarkably consistent. Once the acute overload drops, the nervous system can begin shifting out of constant threat-surveillance and back toward regulation. Integration occurs both in the mind and the body; emotions regulate, allostatic load decreases, and physical symptoms may begin to improve.

When the system has been under strain for a long time, it runs a kind of internal triage. Essential functions take priority, everything else gets pushed aside, and eventually you're running on stress chemistry, rather than genuine energy. Once that pressure lifts, the body starts clearing through the backloost of the time, it's slow and very unglamorous - but the shift is real.

What I've seen clinically is that when survival mode stops running the show, clarity returns in practical ways first. People start sleeping a little deeper. Their digestion settles. The stress spikes aren't as volatile. That's not coincidence, it's the predictable result of the autonomic nervous system finally gaining some space to down-regulate (Porges, 2011). The system stops treating everyday life like an ongoing threat.

Your system also "takes notes" - that's the easiest way to say it in plain language. Long-term stress and emotional load are not metaphorical burdens; the research on allostatic load confirms that the body accumulates the impact over time (McEwen & Wingfield, 2003). When conditions improve, the body starts clearing through that physiological weight. Not instantly. Not neatly. But gradually.

Another thing that became obvious during my integration was how much energy had been going into managing other people's behaviour. When that stops, even briefly, there is often a noticeable release in cognitive load. The prefrontal cortex - the part responsible for planning, reasoning and decision-making - becomes more accessible again (Arnsten, 2009). You start to think more clearly because your brain isn't constantly monitoring the next shock.

From a nervous system perspective, the quiet that emerges during this phase is not "peaceful" in the cliché sense. It's simply the absence of crisis physiology. Once the adrenaline stops running the show, the baseline starts to reveal itself. And that baseline is often much clearer, steadier, and more capable than people expect, especially after years of bracing.

There's also the emotional residue that tends to surface during this stage. Again, not dramatic, it's more a settling of unprocessed strain. The research on trauma recovery consistently shows that regulation comes before insight, not the other way around (Fisher, 2021). Once the body finds some footing, the emotional content becomes manageable, rather than overwhelming.

Grief is common in this phase, and not because the person is "going backwards." It's simply the system having enough stability to process what wasn't safe to feel earlier. Grief for the time spent in overload. Grief for the versions of self that carried too much. Grief for dynamics that had to end so the system could recover. It's not pathology, it's physiology meeting honesty.

One of the most important aspects of integration is that capacity increases. The ventral vagal system - the part responsible for social engagement and grounded presence - becomes more available (Porges, 2011). Decisions become simpler. Boundaries become clearer. Not from defensiveness, but from coherence.

What's most encouraging from a clinical standpoint is that this phase isn't about reinvention. It's about reclamation. The research supports this: once the body is no longer in chronic threat response, people naturally return to their baseline traits, namely competence, clarity, humour and steadiness, the parts that were there long before the chaos (LeDoux, 2015).

Integration is simply the stage where everything finally fits back together, in a way the system can sustain.

# CHAPTER SEVEN

## Integration and Peace

There comes a point where you realise, you're not rebuilding anymore, you're just living. Not performing strength. Not forcing resilience. Just moving through your days without someone else's chaos strapped to your back.

For me, that moment didn't arrive with fireworks. It slipped in quietly, the way steady things do. I noticed it in small ways first: the house felt calm. The animals weren't reacting to stress that wasn't there. My mornings had space in them. My thoughts didn't feel crowded. I wasn't scanning for the next problem to solve. I journalled, painted my nails, listened to music and audiobooks, kept the television off most of the time. I slowly started to manage the back pain. It was a slow, incremental, and steady process. Some days were better than others, but I was so very determined.

Life had shape again.

Not the version I'd planned decades ago, and not the version anyone expected. Just something sturdier, cleaner, more deliberate. I had work that made sense. I had people around me who didn't need managing, decoding, or babying. I had a body that was recovering instead of collapsing. And I had a kind of internal steadiness I'd never experienced before, because I'd never had the conditions for it.

I also realised I was finally dancing to the beat of my own drum - not the clash of unexpected cymbals from elsewhere. There was a rhythm to life that was mine, not dictated, distorted, or disrupted by anyone else's volatility.

The years of navigating narcissistic traits - in childhood, in marriage, in the workplace - had their impact. There's no denying that. But they also sharpened something in me: discernment. The ability to recognise what I will and won't tolerate. The ability to see patterns early. The ability to say no without fear of consequences. And the ability to enjoy the quiet without waiting for it to be taken away.

What surprised me most in this stage was that peace didn't feel foreign. It felt overdue.

You start to understand your own capacity differently here. Not in terms of productivity or endurance, but in terms of coherence. What your system can hold. What it no longer needs to hold. What actually matters. The unnecessary noise drops away, and what's left is a life that feels good.

And sometimes the smallest things turn out to be the biggest markers of healing. For me, one of them was being able to take a long shower - something so ordinary for others, but not for someone who learned early that staying in the shower too long meant the cold water tap in the kitchen would be turned on, scalding my skin and forcing me out. These patterns stay in the body long after the circumstances are gone. You don't even realise they're there until one day you notice you're standing under hot water with no internal countdown, no bracing, no rush. Just taking your time because it's allowed. Because it's safe. Because it's not something reserved for other people anymore.

Another one - a small thing that's actually enormous - is being able to sleep in. For most people, that's nothing. For someone who grew up with the threat of the bed being upended if they didn't get up fast enough - and who even had a bed physically upended in marriage for the same "offence" - sleeping in is its own kind of freedom. It's being able to rest without fear that the ground (or the mattress) will literally be tipped up for you to wake up meeting the floor. That's not a luxury. That's nervous-system safety.

I also found a new kind of purpose here - not in the grand, inspirational sense, but in the practical sense. I had the space to put my experiences, my years in the natural health field, my clinical work, and everything I'd learned about trauma physiology into something that could help others. In a "here's what I've lived, here's what I know, here's what's useful, here's what might ease the load" way.

I've seen enough people carry stress alone. I've seen enough people question themselves because someone else trained them to. I've watched good, competent, kind people shrink themselves to fit inside someone else's dysfunction. Everyone deserves better than that. And I know how heavy that felt for me - and how different it feels when you finally put it down.

That's why this book exists. Not as a retelling of suffering, but as proof that it's possible to walk out the other side intact, informed, and stronger in the places that matter. Not because trauma is "a gift" - I don't subscribe to that. But because clarity, when it finally arrives, is powerful. Post traumatic growth is real.

You don't need to become a different person. You just need the space to become yourself without interference.

And when that happens, when the noise drops, the body settles, and the people around you add to your life rather than drain it, you start to recognise yourself. Not the version shaped by survival, but the one who was always there underneath.

A life reclaimed doesn't look dramatic from the outside. It looks like calm mornings. Work that doesn't hurt. Relationships that feel clean. A body that isn't bracing. The small things that accumulate into something whole.

That's the real ending - and the beginning that follows it.

# Reflections

*Integration, Safety, and the Body's Slow Return to Itself*

By the time someone reaches this stage of their healing, the nervous system has usually spent years - sometimes decades - operating in a heightened, survival-oriented state. When that intensity finally drops, it's not unusual for people to notice that what feels "new" is actually what their baseline was always meant to be. This isn't dramatic; it's biological. Once the stress load reduces, the body adjusts toward what Stephen Porges describes as a more regulated social engagement state, where the system interprets cues as safe, rather than threatening (Porges, 2011).

One of the most common things I see in clinical practice is the way "small" experiences quietly reflect big shifts. The absence of internal bracing. For me it was the long shower. It was being able to choose. These might look minor to the untrained eye, but physiologically, they tell you the system has stopped preparing for impact every waking moment.

When stress has been chronic, the body becomes efficient at predicting threat, even when the threat is historical. This is neuroception in practice: the nervous system assessing risk faster than conscious thought (Porges, 2004). So when someone suddenly notices, "I'm not rushing out of the shower anymore," what they're witnessing is a recalibration of implicit threat detection. The system is receiving enough consistent cues of safety that it no longer anticipates harm.

Sleep is another clear barometer. Difficulty sleeping in, waking abruptly, or feeling restless are well-documented responses to long-term hypervigilance. Research by van der Kolk (2014) demonstrates how bodies conditioned by unpredictable environments often remain alert long after the chaos is gone. Being able to sleep in without an internalised alarm, screaming that consequences are coming, is a sign the nervous system is no longer prioritising protection over rest.

There's also a shift in cognitive load that happens when the body is no longer trapped in survival physiology. Bruce McEwen's work on allostatic load outlines how chronic stress reshapes hormone patterns, inflammation, and executive functioning (McEwen, 2007). When that load reduces, thinking becomes clearer, emotional bandwidth expands, and people often report that they can "hear themselves think" again. It's the brain functioning without constant interruption from stress hormones.

Boundaries also tend to form more naturally here. Not the defensive kind born from fear, but the simple, steady kind that arise when the system has enough regulation to identify what's tolerable and what isn't. Trauma experts such as Janina Fisher note that when hyperarousal decreases, the prefrontal cortex has more capacity for choice, discernment, and self-advocacy (Fisher, 2021). Boundaries aren't born out of bravery - they emerge when the body no longer interprets saying no as dangerous.

Another piece that surfaces in this stage is meaning-making. Not in a spiritual bypass sense, and not in the "everything happens for a reason" framework that can undermine very real harm. Instead, it's the grounded version: once you're out of survival mode, you can look at the accumulation of your learning and ask, "How do I use this in a way that doesn't drain me?" This is a known trajectory in post-traumatic growth literature, where individuals often develop increased insight, clarity, and alignment with personal values - *not* because trauma was beneficial, but because healing allows reorientation (Tedeschi & Calhoun, 2004).

Clinically, this is the phase where people often begin integrating their experiences in a practical, embodied way. They can tolerate calm. They recognise their own needs without guilt. They can discern safe people from unsafe ones, without overriding themselves. Their body gives accurate information again, and they can trust it.

Ultimately, this chapter reflects something essential: healing isn't a single moment. It's a collection of ordinary, almost imperceptible shifts that add up to a life that fits. A life without interference. A life where the nervous system is no longer negotiating with old threats. A life where rest, choice, and groundedness are consistently possible.

Whether someone is rebuilding from a toxic relationship or friendship, a chaotic childhood, or a workplace dynamic that kept them bracing for the next impact, the physiology of recovery follows similar principles: safety, regulation, coherence, and reconnection with one's own internal rhythm.

Your system takes notes - and when those notes finally shift from threat to safety, everything changes.

# CHAPTER EIGHT

# From My Experience to Your Clarity

By the time you reach this point in the book, you will have read my story, and how I healed.

What matters here is an important clarification: I didn't arrive at healing empty-handed. I had decades of professional experience in health, physiology, nutrition and herbal medicine. I understood stress responses. I understood the body and how to support recovery, and I took the time to do exactly that.

Healing wasn't something I stumbled into.
It was something I approached deliberately, systematically, and with respect for what my body had been through.

I was really lucky. I'd been studying this work for so many years, and knew how to rebuild, replenish and restore from the ground up. There was no manual for me to work from, it was about putting together the pieces over time to work out what the best path forward was for me. So from here, part two of my book is about the behaviours, traits, and examples of how they might manifest in different scenarios. In some cases, I've used client examples, and other times I've used my own, to give context on how the behaviours play out.

That distinction and having examples matter to give you context for terms that might be complex.

Many people assume that if you're intelligent, capable, educated, or trained in health, you should immediately see what's happening in a harmful relationship or environment. In reality, narcissistic behaviours don't operate in a straightforward way.

They're often inconsistent, intermittent, and layered with periods of apparent care, charm, or normality. That combination obscures patterns, while you're still navigating them.

This is why the next section of the book exists for you.

Before anyone can begin supporting their body to heal, they need to understand *what they've been responding to.*

The chapters that follow look at:

- The specific behaviours associated with narcissistic traits
- The different presentations or "types" of narcissistic behaviour
- How these behaviours commonly show up in relationships, families, and workplaces
- Why confusion, self-doubt, and physical strain are such consistent consequences.

This isn't about diagnosing people or assigning labels. It's about naming behaviour accurately, so the mind can make sense of what the body has already been carrying.

When behaviour is prolonged, contradictory and destabilising, the body adapts long before conscious understanding catches up. That adaptation can show up as tension, fatigue, pain, gut disturbance, sleep changes, or a constant sense of vigilance - even when you can't yet articulate why.

Understanding the behaviour gives the nervous system context.
Context reduces confusion.
And reduced confusion creates the conditions for recovery.

Once these patterns are clear - not intellectually, but practically so you have clarity, then we can move forward and shift into the physiological supports that help restore balance: nutrients, herbal medicines, and lifestyle protocols that support the body as it returns to steadier ground.

I'm going to give you some information around traits and behaviours, which will help with clarity. This showcases that there are distinct patterns; it's as though they've all got the same playbook, yet they all put their own flair on it. As always, if this is destabilising or triggering for you, please seek the advice of a qualified health care professional.

# PART II

# CHAPTER NINE

## Understanding Narcissistic Behaviour Types and How They Present During Interactions with You

Before we get into the definitions, I want to acknowledge something important: this part of the journey can feel confronting. Sometimes it's the first time the patterns start lining up in a way that actually makes sense, and that realisation can land a little hard, even if it gives clarity. If anything in these descriptions feels familiar, please know you're not meant to walk through this understanding alone. Reaching out to a trusted person, clinician, or support network is always recommended and encouraged.

To understand the patterns you might be recognising, we start with clarity - what these behaviours actually mean. None of these terms are labels for people. They're descriptions of behaviour patterns that show up consistently across research literature.

Why do they do it? Here's two of the reasons.

Number one: you are everything they are not.

Number two: they need you to supply this to them. It's called narcissistic supply.

**Generally, they target strong, capable, empathic people, and once they have you, they need you to maintain a "supply" from you.**

I'll explain further.

A common misconception is that narcissistic behaviour "preys on weak people." That is not what the research shows. In fact, studies consistently find that individuals who attract these patterns often share very specific strengths:

- Empathy
- Warmth
- Emotional generosity
- Conscientiousness
- Loyalty
- Social intelligence
- Competence (practical, emotional, or both).

These qualities make someone **valuable** to a person whose behaviour revolves around:

- Needing admiration
- Wanting emotional labour supplied to them
- Desiring stability they can't generate internally
- Seeking someone who will maintain the relationship even during volatility
- Wanting a partner with skills or attributes they can leverage.

You are not targeted because you are weak. You are targeted because you are **strong in the ways they are not**.

This is not flattery — it's documented in the literature on *narcissistic supply*, interpersonal exploitation, and attachment dynamics (Campbell & Miller, 2011).

Warm, stable people:

- Soothe their volatility
- Make them look good socially

- Offer emotional regulation they cannot generate
- Provide structure
- Offer empathy and patience
- Tolerate inconsistent behaviour longer because they care.

These exact strengths are what make someone vulnerable to manipulative behaviour - not because the strengths are a problem, but because those strengths are *exploited*.

A little more on narcissistic supply.

## Narcissistic Supply

**Narcissistic supply** refers to the **external reinforcement** a person with narcissistic traits relies on to maintain a sense of self-worth, stability, or identity. It is not affection, connection, or genuine intimacy - it's validation that plugs a psychological gap.

In research terms, it describes the **attention, approval, admiration, compliance, or emotional energy** that helps regulate an **unstable or inflated self-concept** (Ronningstam, 2016; Campbell & Miller, 2011).

It can take many forms, including:

- Praise or admiration
- Emotional caretaking
- Agreement or compliance
- Reassurance of their importance
- Someone absorbing their frustration or anger
- Someone tolerating their entitlement, criticism, or volatility.

Importantly:

- **Narcissistic supply is about the *function* the interaction serves for them, not the person providing it.**
- The individual providing the supply is interchangeable from the narcissistic person's perspective - it is the *response* they want, not the relationship.

When supply is abundant, behaviour may appear confident, charming, or settled. When supply is limited or threatened, behaviour often becomes controlling, reactive, or devaluing, as the person works to regain that external stabilisation.

This term is **not a diagnosis** and does not label anyone, including you. It simply describes a pattern identified in the clinical literature explaining why certain behaviours are so inconsistent, confusing and destabilising to others.

What does that mean in the scheme of things? This is was a little hard to get my head around at first, but once I understood it, it becomes very clear, and it gave me an insight into a behaviour that was foreign to me, until I saw it repeatedly in life and in a practice setting.

*When you begin to see and understand the patterns, you can't unsee them. This stands you in very good stead in the future- by seeing it upfront, you are better able to navigate away, and/or set boundaries.*

Let's have a look at what you might experience in an interaction with someone exhibiting narcissistic traits of behaviours, and you might recognise some of these. Then we will move onto the types of narcissism in the hope that you might recognise these.

These terms are becoming more well known in the main stream which means that anyone who has been subject to this kind of behaviour is able to seek support more readily

9.1 Stages of Narcissistic Abuse (Behaviour Patterns) and Terms Used to Describe Them

**Stage 1: Idealisation**

*Love-Bombing or Excessive Admiration*

Intense attention, charm, praise, or support. Your strengths are celebrated, highlighted, and mirrored. They might say things like, you are their soul mate, or they've finally found someone that understands them, or it's like I've known you forever. It feels bonding, validating, and safe. It borders on euphoric because you are literally being 'bombed by love'. A red flag is getting several texts per day when you first meet someone, they become overly familiar too quickly, to get you caught up with them quickly. This is manipulative behaviour at an early stage. They might say they like the same music as you, the same food as you, the same places as you and so on. They make you feel like you've met your dream partner. You might actually feel like you've hit the jackpot, because someone finally 'gets' you. What they do at this stage is mirror your likes, dislikes and behaviours, to create an illusion of "the soul mate".

The intensity feels disproportionate to the stage of the relationship. The defining feature is not kindness - it's *speed* and *excessive intensity* that does not match depth, history, or genuine intimacy.

Research shows that rapid relational intensity can create an accelerated attachment response, making boundaries harder to maintain later on (Strutzenberg & Whisman, 2021).

**Future Faking**

Future faking occurs when someone makes promises, plans, or commitments, with no intention of following through. The "future" becomes a tool - not a shared direction to work towards. They might do this at the start of the relationship, or further down the track, as a way to keep you engaged.

Attachment research notes that false signalling can activate longing, hope, and emotional dependence (Johnson, 2019; Mikulincer & Shaver, 2007).

**Stage 2: Devaluation (Subtle Erosion)**

The tone changes. It's very small remarks at first, which slowly build over time. This can be over weeks, months, or even years. What was once praise, becomes small jabs, then criticism or contempt.
You're told you're "too sensitive," "misunderstanding," or "making things up." They insult what they once admired (or so you thought).

Devaluation is the shift from being idealised to being subtly (or overtly), minimised, dismissed, or diminished. It's not defined by volume - it's defined by *erosion*.

Research on relational instability shows that sudden emotional withdrawal, contempt, or coldness significantly increases stress responses and insecurity (Gottman, 2011; McEwen, 2007).

What creates confusion: You're trying to reconcile the person who admired you, with the behaviour that now hurts you.

**Intermittent Reinforcement**

This is described really well by Dr Ramani Durvasula. The analogy she uses is the slot machines in a casino. They might pay a bit at first, and you keep going back for the reward, because you really want the jackpot, but it doesn't happen and ends up draining your resources. It's also easy to become addicted to, because there's the hope that 'this time' you'll be rewarded. It's sometimes referred to as breadcrumbing.

This is where confusion becomes deeply anchored. Good moments and gestures from the person return just often enough to keep you hoping the "real" version is the idealising one.

This pattern is strongly associated with trauma bonding, because the nervous system becomes locked in a loop of:

- Anticipation
- Relief
- Fear
- Hope
- Disappointment.

The unpredictability itself becomes psychologically binding (Carnell & Lench, 2019).

**What creates confusion:** It's biologically difficult to detach from inconsistent reward cycles.

**Gaslighting and Narrative Distortion**

Gaslighting is the deliberate (or careless, but impactful) distortion of your perception.

Recent work describes gaslighting as a sustained pattern of psychological manipulation that destabilises a person's confidence in their own perception and memory over time, often in the context of intimate or power-imbalanced relationships (Klein, 2023; Klein, Wood, & Bartz, 2025; Darke, 2025; Mento et al., 2023).

Gaslighting is a pattern of communication that undermines your confidence in your own perception, memory, or interpretation of events. Over time, it erodes self-trust.

Studies show gaslighting increases confusion and hypervigilance by destabilising cognitive processing (Sweet, 2019; Durvasula, 2021).

**What Creates Confusion:** Your reality is repeatedly questioned, often with absolute certainty or mockery. It's a form of emotional abuse and manipulation. Over time, self-doubt becomes the default. What this might look like is: "I didn't say that", when you know they did. I had a client who had a partner that repeatedly hid her keys when she needed to go to work and would deny any knowledge. She set up a camera, recorded him hiding them, and he said, "don't be ridiculous, I can't believe you're spying on me" and flipped the narrative. They will alter events, and tell you that you're crazy, or it didn't happen, or change the way the event occurred, so after a while, you doubt your own ability to remember the way things happen. This is very destabilising over time, because you begin to rely on the other person for the 'real story' because you no longer trust your own memory.

They will also rewrite history. I once received a phone call where the person began telling me a completely different story about how a family event went awry, and it was so very far from the truth I had to stop them and say, "I was there, remember?" But there was a time when I would have believed them, and thought my recount was wrong.

**Word Salad, or Circular Conversations**

Word salad refers to communication that is circular, disjointed, tangential, or contradictory, to the point that the conversation becomes impossible to follow. The goal is not clarity - it's disruption. This can be part of any stage, whether it's the devaluation stage or the later discard stage. They usually do this, so they are able to avoid any admission of accountability for their behaviour when you question them or call them out on something,

Exposure to disorganised communication increases cognitive fatigue and reduces the ability to self-advocate (Porges, 2011; van der Kolk, 2014).

Communication research also links unresolved conversational loops to emotional exhaustion and reduced executive functioning (Porges, 2011; McEwen, 2007).

## Triangulation

Triangulation is the use of a third party - real or implied - to create insecurity, comparison, competition, or conflict. It shifts focus away from the person driving the dynamic.

Family systems literature identifies triangulation as a destabilising strategy that increases emotional reactivity (Bowen, 1978; Minuchin, 1974).

## D.A.R.V.O.

(Deny, Attack, Reverse Victim and Offender)

A term coined by Dr. Jennifer Freyd, DARVO describes a defensive pattern used when someone is called out for harmful behaviour:

- **Deny**
- **Attack** the person raising the issue
- **Reverse** the roles so they appear as the
- **Victim**, and you as the
- **Offender.**

This pattern increases confusion and can silence the person seeking clarity (Freyd & Smidt, 2019). You come away from it feeling like you were in the wrong, and it contributes even more to the confusion and self-blame whilst in the relationship. This is exactly what narcissists want. This can happen during any stage of a relationship and can intensify during the devaluation stage.

## Stage 3: Discard or Withdrawal

The discard phase refers to sudden emotional withdrawal, indifference, or abandonment of the relationship, often without explanation. You are either pushed away emotionally, or you disengage out of necessity.

In research terms, it is associated with withdrawal of reinforcement and abrupt relational rupture. It can be because their mask has come off and they know they can't continue with the lie any more, you might finally see them for who are rather than who they pretended to be. Alternatively, they may have found another source of narcissistic supply and they no longer need you for their admiration or emotional caretaking.

This can be abrupt or gradual.

**What creates confusion:** The distance contradicts the earlier intensity, and your nervous system is left with no closure, no coherence, and no explanation.

Relational trauma literature shows that unpredictable relational loss activates survival responses, confusion, and grief responses similar to bereavement (Herman, 2015).

You grieve what you thought the relationship was going to be, but they were never truthful about the relationship from the start, so what you're really grieving is the fantasy they created, and the potential they fed to you, which was not the reality of the relationship. This is really hard, but it gets easier, slowly, incrementally, and with the right help and support of a good health care professional, or a strong support network of people that you know and trust.

## Hoovering and Re-Engagement Attempts

When they leave during the discard phase, or you set a boundary or withdraw, they may suddenly become charming, apologetic, attentive, or emotionally expressive again. They might have discarded you for a new narcissistic supply, and then when it didn't work out, they've sent you a text, or called to see how you are. They can even pretend like nothing has happened and no time has passed. They can also do this after they've intentionally upset you, if they think they've gone too far and you're going to leave, which is not according to their terms on how the relationship is going to play out

This is not always malicious, but it is often patterned.

**What creates confusion:** Just when you gather strength to leave or step back, they shift again.

The cycle of narcissistic abuse:

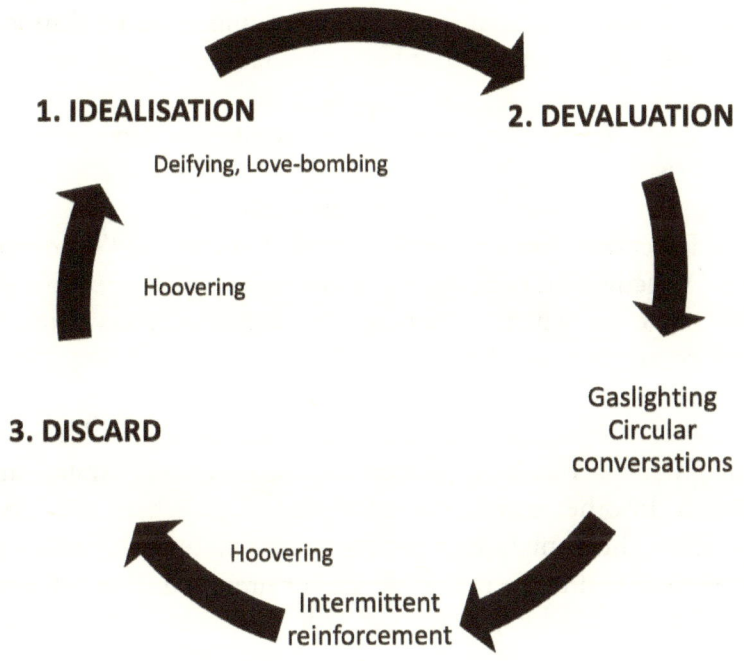

During any of the stages mentioned, you might finally retaliate with a behaviour termed "Reactive Abuse"

## Reactive Abuse

Reactive abuse refers to the intensified, defensive reactions that can emerge after prolonged exposure to destabilising, invalidating, coercive, or hostile behaviour. It is not a personality trait, not an aggression style, and not evidence that someone is "just as bad." It is a stress-driven reaction shaped by accumulated pressure on the nervous system.

Chronic relational stress increases activation of the amygdala and reduces access to the prefrontal cortex, affecting emotional regulation and impulse control (Arnsten, 2009; LeDoux, 2012). Over time, this reduces a person's capacity to respond calmly or flexibly. When the system has been operating in survival mode, even small triggers can push it beyond what it can regulate.

These reactions develop slowly, not suddenly. Environments characterised by coercive control, inconsistency, chronic criticism, or emotional volatility repeatedly activate the body's threat-detection circuits (Stark, 2007; Dutton & Goodman, 2005). As activation persists, the **window of tolerance** narrows - the range in which a person can manage stress without becoming overwhelmed (Siegel, 1999; Ogden et al., 2006).

When that threshold is exceeded, the reaction may look abrupt or heightened, but it is driven by accumulated strain, not intention. In other words, you get to the point where you blow your stack. There might be a tipping point where you've taken it, and taken it, and taken it, and then your limit is reached. This is one of reasons why people will ask themselves, "am I the narcissist?"

Reactive abuse is not equivalent to the behaviours that provoke it.
It is not manipulation, not part of an abusive cycle, and not a

tactic.
It indicates that the nervous system has absorbed more than it can buffer.

Understanding the mechanism helps reduce shame and clarifies why reactions may have felt out of character at the time. Once distance from the destabilising environment is established, reactivity typically decreases as the nervous system may begin to recalibrate (Fisher, 2021; Porges, 2011; van der Kolk, 2014).

Reactive abuse is not pathology - it is the stress-response system exceeding capacity after prolonged interpersonal strain.

THEN THE PATTERN CAN BEGIN ALL OVER AGAIN – STARTING OVER AT THE LOVE-BOMBING PHASE

And you think, "oh there's the person that I first met, maybe we can get back to that again", and you can't blame yourself for thinking that, because they do such a good job during the love-bombing phase…

**Why These Patterns are So Confusing**

These behaviours create destabilisation by blending:

- Kindness with unpredictability
- Warmth with fear
- Clarity with distortion
- Connection with control.

Neurobiologically, unpredictability is a stressor. It disrupts decision-making, increases hypervigilance, and strengthens trauma bonds through intermittent reinforcement (Porges, 2011; McEwen, 2007).

You are not "too sensitive."
Your body and mind responded exactly the way a human nervous system responds to instability.

## 9.2 Types of Narcissistic Behaviour

**None of these categories define a whole person.** They describe patterns of behaviour found consistently in the research, and they help survivors recognise experiences that were confusing or destabilising. This is not about blaming; it is about naming.

People behave in certain ways for complex reasons.

### Grandiose Narcissism

Grandiose narcissism is the form most people recognise first. Research describes it as a pattern of **inflated self-importance, a need for admiration,** and **a tendency to dominate or control conversations and environments** (American Psychiatric Association, 2022). These individuals often present as confident, charming, and capable, particularly in public spaces.

But the confidence is usually brittle. When their sense of superiority is threatened, even slightly, it can flip into defensiveness, contempt, or anger. This response isn't about the person questioning them, it's about protecting their internal balance of dominance and control.

Typical behaviours identified in the research include:

- **Exaggerated achievements** or abilities
- **Strong entitlement** to special treatment
- **Impatience or rage** when challenged
- **Dismissiveness** toward others' needs or expertise
- **A preference for admiration over genuine intimacy.**

These are **behavioural patterns,** not labels for people

## Example

If we look at an example of a client with issues in their professional workplace, there's a pattern that is the same though it will express itself in different ways.

"I've had issues with my boss over the last two years. I went from initially being their golden child, to becoming their scapegoat over a long period of time. I'd witnessed them doing the same thing to other staff members, before it was my turn. They would demean them in front of others in a dramatic way, and they were so convincing, I always thought the other staff members were the issue. One colleague even remarked when it began happening to me, "Oh, so it's your turn now". It's so very difficult when you are discarded, and very confusing. One of my colleagues who had also experienced it, said that it makes you very *wobbly*. I thought that was a good description."

That *"wobbly"* feeling described here is not unusual. When someone alternates between admiration and devaluation, the nervous system can become destabilised. The inconsistency itself creates a kind of psychological disorientation - not because the survivor is weak, but because the human system is designed to seek coherence, predictability, and safety.

This is one of the reasons so many intelligent and capable people feel off-balance in relationships with someone who shows grandiose narcissistic behaviours. It's the *pattern* that destabilises you, not the person being destabilised.

## Vulnerable (Covert) Narcissism

If grandiose narcissism is loud, visible, and self-assured, vulnerable narcissism is its quieter counterpart. The behaviours are different on the surface, but the core mechanisms described in the research are the same: **A fragile sense of self,**

**hypersensitivity to perceived criticism, and a persistent need for external validation** (Pincus & Lukowitsky, 2010).

Where the grandiose style pushes outward, the vulnerable style pulls inward. It can look like:

- **Self-pity or martyr-like positioning**
- **Hyper-reactivity to feedback, even mild feedback**
- **Passive-aggressive behaviour**
- **A strong need for reassurance**
- **Chronic feelings of being unappreciated or misunderstood**
- **Withdrawal or sulking when expectations aren't met.**

The research emphasises that this is *not* shyness, introversion, or low self-esteem.

It's a **defensive system** organised around protecting a fragile sense of self, but done in ways that cause confusion, guilt, and emotional exhaustion for people around them.

Covert narcissistic behaviour often appears in environments where someone feels "less powerful" than the people around them (Dickinson & Pincus, 2003). Instead of asserting dominance directly, they may use:

- Induced guilt
- Quiet sabotage
- Emotional withholding
- Victim-positioning
- Chronic grievances
- *Selective empathy*

## *Selective Empathy* in Narcissistic Behaviour

Research on narcissism and empathy shows a consistent pattern: people high in narcissistic traits often have more difficulty with *emotional* empathy (feeling with another) than with *cognitive* empathy (understanding another's perspective). They may be able to recognise what someone is feeling, but whether they engage with it depends on whether it serves their own needs (Baskin-Sommers et al., 2014; Simard et al., 2023; di Giacomo et al., 2023).

Some clinicians describe this as a kind of **selective empathy** - empathy that is switched on when it is useful (for status, image, or advantage) and switched off when another person's needs clash with their own self-interest (Ronningstam, 2013; Weinberg, 2022).

That doesn't mean "no empathy at all." It means **inconsistent, self-referential empathic engagement**, which fits what many survivors describe, "They could be so kind to others when it made them look good, and so cold to me when I needed support."

Again, these are **behaviours**, not identity labels.

## Heather

Heather grew up in a violent household, with six other brothers and sisters. If any of them misbehaved, her mother would advise her father when he came home from work, and they would be struck with a belt. Her mother was emotionally absent and would often tell the father that Heather had been misbehaving, even when she hadn't. Her mother demanded more help from Heather than the other children, as Heather was the eldest, and her mother became more passive-aggressive towards her (her words) after she reached puberty. As soon as she was old enough to get a job, she found one and moved out. She came to see me a few years later presenting with severe menstrual cramps and pre-menstrual syndrome, that had been non-responsive to the oral contraceptive pill.

This example illustrates a key complexity in understanding vulnerable or covert narcissistic **behaviour: someone can be both a victim in one context and deeply harmful in another.**

Research shows that people who develop vulnerable narcissistic traits may have experienced:

- Chronic helplessness
- Unstable or chaotic environments
- Inconsistent caregiving
- Early trauma or significant losses
- Harsh or unpredictable partners (Kealy & Ogrodniczuk, 2011).

None of these reasons excuse any later behaviour, but it does explain why survivors often hold two truths at the same time:

"I understand where this came from."
and
"It still caused harm."

This duality is often what keeps people confused and emotionally stuck. The behaviour doesn't look like the stereotypical narcissist - there are no grand speeches or obvious arrogance - but the *impact* can still be deeply destabilising.

Vulnerable-style behaviour often leaves people feeling:

- Guilty for having needs
- Responsible for someone else's emotions
- Ashamed for wanting boundaries
- Confused by the swings between fragility and withdrawal
- Worried about triggering emotional collapse.

And like grandiose narcissism, it often creates patterns of:

**self-doubt, chronic second-guessing, and emotional exhaustion** in the people around them.

Clinical and research literature now consistently differentiate between **grandiose** and **vulnerable** narcissism and show that people can move between these states depending on context (Edershile et al., 2020; Mahadevan, 2024; Weinberg, 2022).

## Communal (Benevolent) Narcissism

Communal narcissism can be one of the most confusing forms to recognise because, on the surface, it looks generous, caring, altruistic, and self-sacrificing.

It's the version that says:

"I'm the most helpful one."
"I'm the most supportive friend."
"No one cares as much as I do."

In the research, communal narcissism centres around **grandiosity expressed through "goodness"** rather than achievement or power. Where grandiose narcissism seeks admiration for success, communal narcissism seeks admiration for morality, empathy, helpfulness, or community status (Gebauer et al., 2012).

The behaviour might involve:

- Public displays of helpfulness
- Positioning themselves as the "good one"
- Generosity that increases when others are watching
- Promoting themselves as caring or self-sacrificing
- Using kindness as a bargaining chip
- Withdrawing warmth privately
- Expecting admiration for being virtuous
- Needing validation for their "goodness"
- Becoming defensive or punitive if their moral persona is questioned.

The difficulty for survivors is that the contrast between **public kindness** and **private withdrawal or control** is disorienting.

The confusion itself is a signal.

**Client Example**

A client was in a relationship with someone who was seen as a pillar of the community, very generous with helping people, particularly if they were unwell. At home, though, it was a different story.

This didn't happen immediately, she was love-bombed and the control presented itself slowly over many years. The partner was, in her words, trapped in the 1950s when it came to how the relationship should be, and he wasn't supportive of this woman's need to progress her career, saying that "he knew how men thought, and they were pigs". He wanted her to leave her job because it was 'too stressful for her, and he wanted what was best for her'.

If they went out, he would get angry if another man looked at her, saying he knew what they were thinking, and would then spend the rest of the night in a foul mood. She stopped suggesting they go out together at all. When she had a night planned with her friends, if he was invited, he would pick a fight with her so she would be in a flood of tears beforehand, but as soon as they arrived, he would be happy and charming, as if nothing had happened.

If she was invited to a friend's event without him, he would say that he never sees her and continue complaining, until finally, she would cancel her plans. Then he would go off to bed and leave her on her own for the evening.

Externally, he was friendly, caring and couldn't do enough for people outside the home. Within the home and relationship, she was so very lonely and confused, because the behaviour towards her was quite different to what she experienced in the outside world with him.

## Why this Example Fits Communal Narcissistic Behaviour

This example fits the communal narcissistic pattern. The admiration he sought came from appearing helpful, moral, and supportive **to the outside world**, was very different to his behaviour behind closed doors.

A few key features line up with the literature:

### 1. Public morality as identity

Research shows communal narcissists rely on a *public-facing* image of goodness to feel validated (Gebauer et al., 2012). His reputation as a "pillar of the community" aligns directly with this.

## 2. Outward generosity, inward control

The contrast between external kindness and private withdrawal aligns with evidence that communal narcissism involves **performative helpfulness** rather than genuine empathy (Nehrlich et al., 2019).

## 3. Using "care" as a mechanism of control

Telling her the job was "too stressful" and he wanted "what was best for her" fits the pattern of **benevolent control disguised as concern**. The motive becomes clearer when the "care" restricts autonomy.

## 4. Emotional punishment for independence

Regularly sabotaging her plans, picking fights before events, and withdrawing afterwards, fits the well-established pattern of:

- Controlling access to social support
- De-stabilising the partner's emotional baseline
- Reducing outside connections (American Psychiatric Association, 2022).

## 5. Charm in public, mood volatility in private

This split is strongly associated with narcissistic behaviour — the **public persona** maintained for admiration, and the **private partner** absorbing the instability.

## 6. Confusion in the survivor

Feeling lonely despite being with someone "good" on paper is a hallmark outcome. The research consistently shows that the mismatched behaviour (public warmth vs private dismissal) creates **cognitive disorientation**, especially when the justification is framed as love or protection.

## Malignant Behaviour Patterns

Malignant behavioural patterns sit at the most harmful end of narcissistic traits.

This isn't about someone being self-involved or emotionally inconsistent.
This category reflects behaviour where control, humiliation, and exploitation are used deliberately - often without remorse.

Researchers describe malignant patterns as a **behavioural cluster**, not a diagnosis:

- Targeted cruelty
- Intentional humiliation
- Retaliatory aggression
- Coercive control
- Punishing autonomy
- Lack of empathy or remorse
- Willingness to harm someone psychologically or physically to maintain dominance
  (Miller et al., 2010; APA, 2022; Dutton, 2007).

It's where narcissistic antagonism overlaps with psychopathic features.

**Not everyone who behaves badly belongs in this category.**
But certain actions map cleanly onto what the literature describes.

### Key Features in the Research

### 1. Punitive Aggression

Harm is used as punishment - for disobedience, independence, or perceived disrespect.

### 2. Coercive Control

Limiting freedom, autonomy, access to resources, or safety. Coercive control is now recognised as a patterned form of abuse where one person uses a range of behaviours - isolation, monitoring, humiliation, financial restriction, threats - to dominate another and erode their autonomy (AIHW, 2022; MacDonald, 2020; Fitz-Gibbon et al., 2024).

Emerging work also links higher levels of pathological narcissism with increased use of coercive control tactics, in intimate relationships (Day et al., 2025)

**3. Humiliation as a Tactic**

Public or private "jokes," pranks, or staged moments that degrade the partner.

**4. Exploitative Manipulation**

Using another person's vulnerability or trust against them.

**5. Emotional Indifference to Harm**

No remorse, or an attempt to minimise, mock, or blame the target.

These patterns are documented across the coercive control literature (Stark, 2007; Follingstad, 1990) and narcissistic aggression research (Reidy et al., 2008).

**Examples**

**1. Public Humiliation**

"This woman experienced a humiliating situation at a wedding where her husband offered to catch her in the style of "Dirty Dancing" the way Patrick Swayze catches Jennifer Grey at the end of the movie. The song from the movie was playing as the night was drawing to a close.

She agreed, took a run up, and launched herself toward her husband to catch her over this head. He stepped out of the way at the last second, and she fell to the ground. The other guests gasped and ran to her aid because she was fully winded, and he stood there laughing, saying 'it was a joke, stop over-reacting'.

When confronted by another guest, he dismissed them and went off to get a drink. When she tried to speak to him about it the next morning, he said, "Why do you have to make such a big deal of everything? There you go again, bringing up the past."

### This Fits the Pattern

This is **humiliation framed as humour**, delivered publicly, with:

- Intentional setup
- Deliberate withdrawal of support
- Social degradation
- Mockery afterward
- Reframing her distress as overreaction.

This kind of tactic is widely recorded in malignant behavioural clusters (Reidy et al., 2008; Follingstad et al., 1990). There is a clear intent-to-dominance, wrapped in a "joke."

### 2. Being Upended Out of Bed

A client conveyed to me that if they slept in too late, their partner used to go into the bedroom shouting out "Get up! Get up! Get up!" Also on one occasion, when she was exhausted from work, studying and raising children, she had overslept, and her husband upended the bed. She fell onto the floor while she was still asleep. This also fits the pattern.

- **Punitive aggression** (punishment for sleeping "too long")
- **Intentional fear induction**
- **Physical dominance**
- **No concern for harm**
- **Disproportionate reaction**
- **Destruction of basic safety in a place of rest.**

This maps directly onto coercive control literature describing "forced destabilisation" and "physical intimidation as behavioural correction" (Stark, 2007).

These two examples illustrate two **different expressions** of malignant behaviour:

1. Public humiliation framed as a joke
2. Private aggression framed as "teaching you a lesson"

They are not repeated actions.
They are **one-off acts,** which is common - malignant behaviour doesn't need repetition to make its impact.
Single events can lodge deeply in the nervous system because of the **surprise, humiliation, and the collapse of safety** they create.

Both examples meet criteria across multiple research models:

- **Coercive control tactics**
- **Sadistic humour or humiliation**
- **Punitive physical aggression**
- **Lack of empathy**
- **Justification after harm.**

## Machiavellian Behaviour

Machiavellian behaviour is its own category in the research literature.

It's not loud, emotional, or explosive.
It's calculated.

Where narcissistic behaviour often centres around **needing admiration, protecting ego, or reacting to perceived threats**, Machiavellian behaviour is grounded in:

- **Planned manipulation**
- **Long-game strategy**
- **Instrumental charm**
- **Cold, deliberate decision-making**
- **A focus on personal gain over connection**
- **A willingness to exploit if it serves a goal.**

The difference matters:

- A narcissistic person reacts because their ego is threatened.
- A Machiavellian person acts because it benefits them.
- And someone with **both** traits can do significant harm because the emotional volatility of narcissism meets the strategic detachment of Machiavellianism (Jones & Paulhus, 2014).

Machiavellian behaviour tends to be:

## 1. Calculated, not reactive

They plan.
They position.
They gather information that can be used later.

## 2. Subtle and socially intelligent

This is the person who understands how to play a room without needing applause.

## 3. Outcome-driven

Relationships are transactions.
People are resources.
Every choice serves a purpose.

## 4. Less concerned with image than narcissistic behaviour

A narcissistic person needs to *look good*.
A Machiavellian person needs to *win*.
If looking bad helps them win, they'll tolerate it.

## 5. Overlaps with narcissistic behaviour

Both involve manipulation, but for different reasons:

- Narcissistic manipulation protects ego or image
- Machiavellian manipulation serves strategy or advantage.

This is why some people who survive narcissistic abuse feel an uncanny sense of "calculated coldness" underneath certain actions.
That layer is Machiavellian, not narcissistic.

## 6. In the research literature

Machiavellianism is classified as part of the Dark Triad (Paulhus & Williams, 2002):

- **Narcissism** (grandiosity, entitlement, ego-reactivity)
- **Machiavellianism** (strategic manipulation, emotional detachment)
- **Psychopathy** (low empathy, impulsivity, aggression).

Dr. Ramani Durvasula extends this into the **Dark Tetrad** with the addition of **sadism**, because cruelty for pleasure shows up too frequently to ignore in abusive relationships.

Machiavellian behaviour sits right in the middle: *strategic, cold, and quietly harmful.*

### Research-Based Example of Machiavellian Behaviour

### Evidence-Based Example (from Academic Research)

One of the clearest illustrations of Machiavellian behaviour in the research literature comes from controlled experiments on strategic interpersonal manipulation (Jones & Paulhus, 2009). In these studies, individuals who scored high on Machiavellianism consistently used **calculated, unemotional tactics** to secure the best outcome for themselves, even when cooperation would have benefited everyone involved.

For example, in negotiation simulations where participants had the option to collaborate or compete, high-Machiavellian individuals were far more likely to:

- Withhold information intentionally
- Feign cooperation to extract details from others
- Switch strategies at the last moment
- Leave their counterpart disadvantaged

The behaviour wasn't reactive.
It wasn't emotional.
It wasn't driven by insecurity or a need to look good.

It was strategic.

The goal was to **maximise their gain**, even if it meant betraying someone who believed they were working together. They remained calm, controlled, and focused, not because they were grounded, but because emotional neutrality served the strategy.

Researchers describe this as "instrumental exploitation"- using another person as a tool to achieve an outcome (Jones & Paulhus, 2011).

It's the opposite of impulsive cruelty, and very different from ego-driven conflict.

**Why this Example is Useful for You**

This kind of behaviour often feels confusing if you've been on the receiving end of it.
It's subtle.
It's planned.
And it can be mistaken for intelligence, or even leadership at first.

The harm comes from the fact that: You're not interacting with someone who is emotionally dysregulated. You're interacting with someone who is **deliberately managing the impression they give you,** while quietly arranging the outcome that benefits them alone.

There's no blow-up.
No shouting.
No dramatic episodes.

Just someone playing a long game, you didn't know you were in.

This is why Machiavellian patterns can sit quietly underneath other behaviours - and why, when combined with narcissistic traits, they can be especially destabilising.

**References (for the example above)**

Jones, D. N., & Paulhus, D. L. (2009). Machiavellianism. In M. R. Leary & R. H. Hoyle (Eds.), *Handbook of individual differences in social behavior* (pp. 93–108). Guilford Press.

Jones, D. N., & Paulhus, D. L. (2011). The role of impulsivity in the Dark Triad of personality. *Personality and Individual Differences, 51*(5), 679–682.

Paulhus, D. L., & Williams, K. M. (2002). The Dark Triad of personality: Narcissism, Machiavellianism, and psychopathy. *Journal of Research in Personality, 36*(6), 556–563.

## 9.3 Why People Feel So Confused After Experiencing Narcissistic Behaviours

Confusion is one of the most consistent after-effects of narcissistic behaviour. Even the most grounded, capable, intelligent people describe a kind of fog, not because they're weak or naïve, but because the behaviour itself is designed to destabilise.

That is why clarity is so important here: Your confusion does not mean you "missed the signs." It means the behaviour was strategic, inconsistent and disorienting by design.

### Why the Nervous System Struggles to Make Sense of Narcissistic Abuse

When a relationship swings between comfort and threat, the nervous system becomes disoriented.

Here's the simple version:

- When someone is warm → your system opens
- When someone is cold or aggressive → your system protects
- When someone cycles unpredictably → your system gets stuck in hypervigilance

This isn't weakness.
This is biology.

Unpredictability is one of the strongest triggers for stress activation (Porges, 2011; LeDoux, 2012).

Your system tries to solve the puzzle, hoping that clarity will lead to safety.

But in narcissistic abuse, the puzzle has no consistent rules.

When You Still Miss Them

It's common to miss:

- The version of them who showed care
- The promise of who you thought they were
- The connection you hoped was real
- The stability you were trying to build
- The meaning you gave the relationship.

Nothing about that is shameful, it is human.

You bonded with the parts of them that felt warm, close, or hopeful - and your brain learned to expect those parts to return.

The confusion is by no means a flaw, it's a normal response to inconsistent behaviour.

**Why Narcissistic Abuse Feels So Personal - But Isn't**

Their behaviour reflects their patterns, not your worth. If you had been:

- Colder
- Less empathetic
- Less grounded
- Less capable
- Less loving

- you simply would not have been useful to them.

Your qualities were the drawcard.
Not your weaknesses.

# A Note for You

Before you move to the next chapter, just take a breath.

If any part of this section stirred something in you, it's your system responding to information that finally makes sense. You're allowed to take this slowly. You're allowed to pause. And you're absolutely allowed to reach out for support rather than try to shoulder all of this on your own.

What I hear more often than not is, "So it's not me?" "I wasn't the issue?" "You mean it's a distinct pattern?" No, it was never you, you weren't the issue, and yes, it's a distinct pattern.

Understanding the patterns is about giving yourself clarity where there was fog. It was never your fault, and knowing how these behaviours operate, is like opening a window to let the fresh air in.

# CHAPTER TEN

# Behaviour Clusters that Destabilise

Before moving into healing, it's important for you to understand the behavioural patterns that appear consistently in narcissistic relational dynamics across research literature. None of these terms are labels for people. They describe **documented behaviour patterns** - behaviours that can emerge in relationships, families, workplaces, friendships, and community settings.

A gentle reminder: Understanding these patterns can feel confronting. This is not work to do alone. It is always wise to reach out to a therapist, trusted professional, or support person if this material brings up any discomfort or memories.

## 10.1 - Behaviour Cluster Overview

Researchers have repeatedly found that narcissistic behavioural patterns tend to group into broad functional clusters rather than appearing in a strict sequence (Campbell & Miller, 2011; Pincus et al., 2009).

Using clusters helps readers understand *why* certain interactions feel destabilising, rather than getting lost in the details.

The four major clusters are:

1. Bonding Behaviours

Love bombing
Future faking

## 2. Destabilisation Behaviours

Gaslighting
Word salad
Triangulation
Circular conversations

## 3. Control Behaviours

Devaluation
DARVO

## 4. Exit Behaviours

Discard
Hoovering

These clusters often overlap. They do not always appear in a neat order. The overall impact is cumulative, rather than linear.

### 10.1.1 - Bonding Behaviours

Bonding behaviours are designed to build closeness quickly. They may feel intoxicating, intense, or unusually fast-paced.

**Love Bombing**

Love bombing is the rapid flooding of attention, praise, affection, promises, intensity, or future-oriented fantasies at the beginning of a relationship (Durvasula, 2021). It creates a heightened emotional state that can make later inconsistencies harder to identify.

**Future Faking**

Future faking refers to promises about the future that create attachment, but are never fulfilled (Durvasula, 2021). The intent isn't long-term follow-through, it's immediate emotional influence.

### 10.1.2 - Destabilisation Behaviours

These behaviours create confusion, self-doubt, and emotional disorientation.

### Gaslighting

Gaslighting occurs when someone intentionally or consistently dismisses, distorts, or denies your lived experience (Sweet, 2019). It makes you question your memory, perception, or reality.

### Word Salad

Word salad involves long, circular, or tangential responses that prevent resolution of an issue (Durvasula, 2021). It creates exhaustion, not clarity.

### Triangulation

Triangulation occurs when a third person - real, named, or actively recruited - is brought into the dynamic to create tension, rivalry, or insecurity (Campbell & Miller, 2011).

It can sound like:

- "Everyone agrees with me."
- "Other people think you're being unreasonable."
- "So-and-so understands me better."

Triangulation is common in:

- Families
- Romantic partnerships

- Sibling dynamics
- Friendship groups
- Workplace teams
- Peer circles.

Sometimes the third person is fully aware of being included. Sometimes they don't realise they are being used to increase pressure or diminish your credibility.

The aim is the same: shifting the power balance, altering the emotional tone, and destabilising direct communication.

## Circular Conversations

Circular conversations involve going around the same topic repeatedly without resolution (Streep, 2019). The goal is not understanding - it's delay, confusion and emotional fatigue.

## 10.1.3 - Control Behaviours

These behaviours maintain dominance through criticism, blame, or reversal.

## Devaluation

Devaluation is the shift from idealisation to criticism, withdrawal, contempt, or emotional coldness (Ronningstam, 2016). It is often inconsistent, which heightens confusion.

## DARVO

DARVO stands for:

- **Deny** the behaviour
- **Attack** the person confronting it
- **Reverse Victim and Offender** roles (Freyd, 1997).

This pattern is well-documented in interpersonal violence research.
It can leave a person shocked at how quickly a simple concern becomes an accusation turned back onto them.

### 10.1.4 - Exit Behaviours

### Discard

Discard refers to abrupt withdrawal, distancing, or abandonment - emotional or literal, often without explanation (Durvasula, 2021).
It may happen after a period of devaluation or simply when the relationship no longer serves the individual's needs.

### Hoovering

Hoovering is any attempt to re-engage after a period of distance, often using promises, nostalgia, guilt, or manipulation (Streep, 2019).
The intention is not reconnection - it's re-access.

### Why These Behaviours Create Confusion

Confusion after narcissistic abuse is expected, it is not a sign of weakness.
Neurobiological research shows that inconsistent behaviour activates survival mechanisms, keeps the nervous system in hypervigilance, and interferes with clear decision-making.

Three core mechanisms contribute:

1. Intermittent Reinforcement

When positive and negative behaviours alternate unpredictably, attachment intensifies (Ferster & Skinner, 1957).

2. Cognitive Dissonance

When someone's words do not align with their actions, the mind strains to reconcile the contradiction (Hinojosa et al., 2017).

3. Survival Physiology

The nervous system learns to anticipate threat, even in calm moments (Porges, 2011).

None of this is your fault.

These are predictable human responses to inconsistent or destabilising relational environments.

**Integration of Behaviour Clusters**

The clusters aren't linear stages.
They move, blend, overlap, and shift depending on context.

Understanding them gives you:

- Language for confusing experiences
- Clarity about what actually happened
- A sense that they're not "crazy," "dramatic," or "overreacting"
- A starting point for reclaiming agency.

And most importantly: **an understanding that these reactions were normal responses to abnormal behaviour patterns.**

# CHAPTER ELEVEN

# The Disengagement: When the Pattern Ends Abruptly

Abrupt withdrawal in a relationship marked by unpredictability or controlling behaviour can create a distinct physiological and psychological response. Researchers in trauma, attachment and stress physiology, have documented that sudden relational rupture often activates the body's threat-detection systems, particularly when the relationship has involved cycles of inconsistency or conflict (Fisher, 2021; Porges, 2011; McEwen, 2007).

This chapter explains **what happens inside the body and mind** during an abrupt end to a difficult relational pattern. It is written so you can understand the mechanisms, rather than personalise the material.

There is no pathologising, no diagnostic implication, and no assumption about what you've lived through.

### 1. Abrupt Relational Rupture as a Stressor

Research shows that sudden loss of predictability in a close relational system activates the sympathetic nervous system — the body's instinctive "threat readiness" response (LeDoux, 2020; Porges, 2011).

This may include:

- Increased heart rate
- Muscle tension
- Shallow breathing

- Sleep disruption
- Heightened startle response.

This is a biological pattern, not a reflection of emotional weakness.
When familiar cues - even stressful ones - are suddenly removed, the nervous system must rapidly recalibrate its sense of safety.

## 2. Loss of Predictability and the Brain's Response

Predictability is an important regulatory anchor for the nervous system (Porges, 2011).
Abrupt changes in relational patterns -including withdrawal, silence, distancing, or severing contact -interrupt that anchor.

This can activate:

a) The Amygdala (Threat Detection)

The amygdala becomes more active when the brain cannot forecast what will happen next (Pessoa, 2018). This increase in activity is linked with:

- Hypervigilance
- Scanning for danger
- Difficulty concentrating.

b) The Prefrontal Cortex (Reasoning and Planning)

During high stress, the prefrontal cortex's ability to organise thoughts or plan can temporarily decrease (Arnsten, 2009). This can create difficulty making decisions or settling the mind.

c) The Default Mode Network (Self-Referential Processing)

Research shows that during major relational disruption, the brain may shift into increased self-referential processing (Barrett, 2017).

# Life After Narcissists

This can contribute to internal questioning or repeated thoughts about what occurred.

These responses are **documented neural patterns,** rather than interpretations of your internal world.

3. Cognitive Dissonance During Abrupt Disengagement

Cognitive dissonance occurs when conflicting information is held at the same time -particularly when words and actions do not align (Hinojosa et al., 2017). When a relationship has involved inconsistency, the sudden withdrawal of communication or connection can intensify this strain.

This is not describing your emotions. It is a description of how the brain attempts to resolve incompatible signals.

Common documented effects include:

- Mental "looping" as the brain searches for coherence
- Difficulty letting go of unanswered questions
- Physiological tension while trying to reconcile contradictory experiences.

These experiences reflect the brain's effort to restore equilibrium, they are not a personal failing.

4. Shame as a Neurobiological Response

In the context of relational disruption, shame is frequently observed as a stress-based cognitive response, not a moral judgment (Moll et al., 2008; Tangney & Dearing, 2002).

Shame in this context is associated with:

- Increased activity in brain regions tied to self-evaluation

- Uncertainty about social belonging
- Heightened threat awareness.

This is a *documented pattern*, not a prediction.

This is to let you know: shame in relational rupture is a biological stress response, not an indicator of fault.

5. Allostatic Load and the "Final Stressor" Concept

Allostatic load refers to the cumulative physiological "wear and tear" from prolonged stress (McEwen, 2007). Research shows that when the body has been sustaining stress for a long period, a final stressor -even a minor one- can trigger an amplified reaction.

This is not an assumption that you've endured long-term stress. It simply explains the mechanism:

- Prolonged activation of stress hormones
- Reduced capacity for new stress
- Intensified response when unpredictability spikes suddenly.

Understanding this can help separate **physiology from interpretation**.

6. The Sudden Silence: Why the Nervous System Reacts

An abrupt end to a stressful relational dynamic removes familiar cues, even cues that were difficult to endure. Stress physiology research shows that the nervous system relies on patterned cues to maintain orientation (Porges, 2011).

When those cues disappear quickly, the body may register:

- Uncertainty
- Heightened scanning

- Difficulty settling.

This is not a sign the relationship was healthy. It is the nervous system shifting from one pattern to an unanticipated absence of pattern.

7. Documented Emotional and Physical Reactions

Literature notes common reactions people *can* experience during abrupt relational rupture.
These are not predictions; they are simply research-based possibilities:

- Increased stress hormones (Caine et al., 2020)
- Sleep disruption
- Intrusive thoughts
- Loss of appetite or increased appetite
- Restlessness
- Low mood
- Irritability.

These reactions are tied to neural and hormonal shifts, not character traits.

8. Why Understanding the Physiology Helps

When a confusing or stressful relational pattern ends abruptly, understanding the neurobiology:

- Reduces self-blame
- Provides structure for what can otherwise feel chaotic
- Supports informed decision-making
- Reinforces that physiological responses are normal human patterns.

This chapter is not offering advice.
It is providing a **framework** so you can recognise that there is a

clear, grounded explanation for the reactions documented in the literature.

# CHAPTER TWELVE

# Why Clarity Comes After Distance

There's a particular kind of understanding that only arrives when you're finally out of the situation. Not because you "should have seen it earlier," and not because you missed something obvious. Clarity needs space. It can't form properly when you're bracing, compensating, apologising, calming things down, or trying to hold everything together.

Distance gives you that space.

For many people, the real understanding begins **after** the environment is quiet, their body steadies, and their mind can finally process what has been happening without interruption. This chapter explains why that happens - physiologically, psychologically, and emotionally - so you can take in your own insights without judgement or self-criticism.

### 1. Distance Lets Your Nervous System Settle

When the unpredictable behaviour stops - whether that was rage, criticism, silent treatment, volatility, or ongoing tension - your nervous system finally gets a chance to down-shift.

Research has shown that chronic interpersonal stress keeps the amygdala activated (LeDoux, 2012), narrows your attention onto threat cues, and dials down the prefrontal cortex (Arnsten, 2009). You're not thinking clearly because your brain isn't supposed to think clearly under threat. It's supposed to protect you.

When you step away:

- The stress hormones reduce
- The survival circuitry eases
- The thinking part of the brain starts coming back online.

This is often the first time you can look at events without feeling overwhelmed by them.

## 2. Your Cognitive Bandwidth Returns

High-stress environments consume the mental resources required for:

- Reflection
- Reasoning
- Decision-making
- Self-observation
- Perspective-taking.

When you're living inside the situation, that space isn't available. Your mind is too busy trying to prevent escalation, track mood changes, keep the peace, or avoid conflict. It's survival, not clarity.

Once you have distance, the cognitive load drops. You have the bandwidth to examine what happened, piece things together, and understand the dynamics without feeling like you're drowning in them.

## 3. Your Internal Cues Reappear

Prolonged exposure to blame, criticism, or denial can dull your internal signals. People begin doubting themselves, dismissing their instincts, and second-guessing their perceptions. It's not a personal flaw, it's adaptation.

When the external pressure is removed, your internal cues start resurfacing:

- "That wasn't okay."
- "I ignored that at the time."
- "I can see the pattern now."
- "That comment was minimising."

These insights don't show up during the chaos. They show up in the calm that follows it. Your system simply couldn't afford to be insightful earlier; it was too busy trying to keep you safe.

### 4. The Cognitive Dissonance Reduces

Inside the situation, you're constantly managing conflicting information:

- "They say they care, but their behaviour is cruel."
- "They say they're sorry, but nothing changes."
- "They blame me, but the reaction doesn't match anything I did."
- "They say I'm the problem, but no one else treats me this way."

This is cognitive dissonance - the mental strain of trying to reconcile incompatible things at once (Hinojosa et al., 2017).

Distance removes the contradictions. There's no new behaviour arriving to override or confuse your insights. Your mind stops wrestling with the "version of events" you were given and is finally able to accept the reality of what occurred.

### 5. Safety Allows Accurate Perspective

When you're no longer walking on eggshells, waiting for the next shift in tone, or monitoring someone's reactions, your entire system recalibrates. Safety gives you access to information you previously had to block out because acknowledging it was too threatening - emotionally or physically.

People often say:

- "I didn't realise how exhausted I was."
- "I didn't see how much I'd adapted."
- "I didn't understand the extent of it until I got out."
- "Only now can I connect the dots."

This isn't hindsight bias.
It's the brain finally having the capacity to process reality.

## 6. Insight Is No Longer Interrupted

During the relationship, any moment of clarity usually gets overridden:

- By charm
- By crying
- By anger
- By denial
- By promises
- By minimisation
- By blame
- By emotional collapse
- By silence
- By attention withdrawal.

There is no space for your insight to consolidate.

Once you have distance, nobody interrupts your internal process. The insight stays intact long enough for you to recognise it, name it, and trust it.

## 7. Why You Didn't See It Earlier

People often feel ashamed that they "didn't see the signs," but this shame isn't warranted. When someone is:

- Stressed
- Overwhelmed
- Criticised

- Confused
- Trying to keep the peace
- Adjusting to the other person's reactions
- Responsible for children or family
- Financially dependent
- Traumatised
- Hopeful for change.

The brain does not analyse. It copes.

The timing of your clarity doesn't reflect your intelligence, strength, or capability. It reflects the moment your nervous system finally had the capacity to process what was happening.

## 8. Your System Begins to Regulate

This stage often feels strange because it's unfamiliar, not because something is wrong.

You may notice:

- Improved sleep
- More stable energy
- Less hypervigilance
- The ability to rest
- Clearer decision-making
- Softer internal pressure
- Fewer stress-related symptoms.

This is the return of your actual baseline - the one you couldn't access under constant stress.

"Clarity doesn't arrive in the middle of chaos. It comes when your body finally feels safe enough to let the truth land. If your understanding is only emerging now, that's not a failure - it's timing. Your system is doing exactly what human systems do. You're allowed to take this in at your own pace."

# Reflections

When you step out of an environment marked by inconsistency, criticism, volatility, or emotional instability, the body and mind don't immediately "feel clear." What most people notice first is the absence of pressure - and only then does the understanding begin to unfold. These reflections explain **why clarity emerges after distance**, strictly through evidence-based mechanisms.

1. The Nervous System Needs Safety Before Insight is Possible

When you're under chronic interpersonal stress, the brain prioritises survival, not analysis. Research has shown that repeated emotional unpredictability activates the amygdala - the brain's threat-detection centre - and reduces the functional capacity of the prefrontal cortex (Arnsten, 2009; LeDoux, 2012).

This affects:

- Planning
- Reasoning
- Impulse control
- Ability to reflect
- Ability to think in a linear way.

Once distance is established, sympathetic activation begins to settle and the parasympathetic system becomes more accessible. You are not "finally seeing clearly because you should have known earlier." You are seeing clearly because the part of the brain required for insight is finally able to function.

2. Cognitive Load Reduces and Processing Returns

Chronic stress increases allostatic load - the cumulative wear on the body from repeated stress responses (McEwen & McEwen, 2017).
When someone is constantly adjusting to another person's behaviours, moods, or reactions, their cognitive resources become tied up in monitoring and managing interactions.

Distance reduces this load. With fewer demands on attention, the mind naturally begins to organise information that couldn't be organised before. This isn't "overanalysis"; it is simply cognitive capacity returning.

3. Internal Cues Re-Activate When External Pressure Stops

Research in trauma psychology shows that ongoing relational stress can suppress interoceptive awareness (Fisher, 2021). Interoception is the ability to sense what you feel inside your own body. When the environment is unpredictable, many people learn to override their instincts because responding to the external situation becomes more important than internal cues.

After distance, internal signals begin to strengthen again:

- Recognising discomfort
- Understanding boundaries
- Noticing patterns
- Identifying behaviours that weren't visible under stress.

This is not "dwelling on the past."
It is the nervous system restoring access to information that was previously suppressed to keep you functioning.

4. Reduced Exposure Means Reduced Dissonance

Cognitive dissonance is the psychological tension created when someone's actions and words do not align (Hinojosa et al., 2017). During the relationship, every moment of dissonance is often followed by an interruption: a justification, a denial, a promise, or another behaviour that overrides the uncomfortable insight.

Distance stops the interruptions. Without new contradictory messages arriving, the mind can process events without competing versions of reality. The dissonance reduces because the conflicting input reduces.

5. Safety Restores Perspective

Research on relational trauma shows that accurate self-observation requires emotional safety (Porges, 2011). When safety increases, the nervous system shifts from defence to regulation. This creates space for perspective-taking, something not possible during chronic activation.

People often interpret this delayed understanding as a personal failure.
It is not.
It reflects the reality that the brain only integrates information when the environment is no longer threatening.

**I call it the "what the fuck just happened" moment - that point where the truth becomes visible because your system is no longer under siege.**

6. Integration is a Physiological Response, Not a Moral One

Post-stress clarity is a physiological process driven by:

- Reduction in cortisol (Doane et al., 2015)
- Restored prefrontal cortex activity (Arnsten, 2009)
- Decreased limbic reactivity (LeDoux, 2012)
- Improved interoception (Fisher, 2021)
- Increased autonomic regulation (Porges, 2011).

This is why clarity appears *after* the threat has passed - not during it.

Nothing about delayed clarity indicates weakness, naivety, or lack of intelligence.
It reflects neurobiology.

**Small things will float up, and you'll realise the smoke and mirrors are no longer in play - that's when the capacity for clarity emerges.**

Clarity arriving later is by no means a failure, and sometimes it comes with the idea, "why didn't I see it before?" You can't see it when you're in it. The amygdala in your brain had taken over to keep you safe, and the pre-frontal cortex in your brain, which governs reasoning had to take a back step while that was happening.
When the body finally has enough safety to let the truth make sense, it is a sign of recovery, not regret, and should be celebrated.

# CHAPTER THIRTEEN

**The Stabilisation Phase**

Leaving a destabilising environment doesn't deliver instant clarity or emotional certainty. Stabilisation begins in the body first. It is quieter, slower, and a lot more physical than people often expect. This chapter outlines what stabilisation actually looks like - without romanticising it or framing it as a sudden turning point.

Stabilisation is the body's first priority.
Your biology recalibrates before your emotions do.
It isn't a setback - it's your system catching its breath.

**1. Physiological Stabilisation**

*What the body starts doing automatically when the environment no longer requires constant vigilance.*

1.1 The threat response begins to stand down

Prolonged exposure to inconsistent, volatile, or critical behaviour keeps the nervous system in a state of chronic activation. Research shows that under ongoing interpersonal stress, the amygdala becomes more reactive while the prefrontal cortex - responsible for planning, reasoning, and decision-making - becomes less accessible (Arnsten, 2009; LeDoux, 2012).

Once the source of stress is no longer present, the threat response doesn't shut off all at once. It reduces gradually as the body recognises that the demand has changed.

People may notice physical shifts such as:

- Steadier breathing
- Reduced muscle tension
- Fewer stress-driven physical reactions
- A decrease in startle responses.

These changes reflect the nervous system adjusting to the absence of ongoing disruption.
They're physiological recalibrations, not emotional conclusions.

1.2 Cortisol begins to regulate

Chronic relational stress elevates cortisol over time, contributing to allostatic load - the wear and tear on the body from repeated stress activation (McEwen & McEwen, 2017). Distance allows this system to downshift.

Some benefits may be:

- Waking up less exhausted
- Fewer cortisol-driven spikes early in the morning
- Steadier energy throughout the day
- Less internal jitteriness.

This doesn't mean the stress response has "finished." It means the endocrine system finally has room to self-correct.

1.3 Digestion reawakens

The GI tract is one of the first areas affected by stress. Sympathetic activation slows digestion, alters motility, and can disrupt appetite.

Once the system begins stabilising, changes may include:

- Appetite returning in stages
- Fewer stress-related Gastro-intestinal symptoms
- More consistent bowel function.

These improvements reflect increased vagal influence -the parasympathetic processes associated with safety (Porges, 2011).

1.4 Sleep recalibrates – Gradually

Sleep rarely improves in a straight line.

Early stabilisation may include:

- Deeper sleep occurring intermittently
- Occasional extended sleep periods
- Difficulty initiating sleep despite tiredness
- Vivid or stress-related dreams
- Fluctuations in sleep quality.

These variations reflect the brain reprocessing information that previously had no safe context.

Your brain does some overdue housekeeping, but it's not always tidy.

1.5 Clarity windows appear - Then fade

Stabilisation often brings small, brief moments of recognition:

- "That behaviour wasn't normal."
- "That reaction makes sense now."
- "I'm breathing differently."

These short windows are followed by foggier periods.
This oscillation is normal.
It reflects a nervous system shifting between activation and recovery.

## 2. Emotional Stabilisation

*Why emotional responses may feel inconsistent during early recovery.*

2.1 Emotional flattening is a normal transition

After prolonged stress, emotional processing systems often move into conservation mode.

This is not pathology - it is efficiency.

Research shows that systems under chronic strain require time to recalibrate once the immediate stress has reduced (Fisher, 2021).

Common experiences include:

- Emotional quietness
- Detachment
- Neutrality
- A temporary sense of blankness.

This is stabilisation, not regression.

## 2.2 Delayed emotions are expected

As stress hormones decrease, the body becomes capable of accessing emotions that previously had no room to surface.

Tears appearing weeks or months later is common.
It's not "late grief."
It's accessible grief.

## 2.3 The system may not register calm as familiar

When unpredictability has been a long-term baseline, a calmer environment can actually feel unfamiliar.
This isn't a psychological failing.
It is conditioned neuroception - the nervous system's automatic evaluation of safety (Porges, 2011).

## 2.4 Relief and loneliness can coexist

It is common for stabilisation to involve mixed states such as:

- Relief
- Loneliness
- Anger
- Sadness
- Gratitude
- Emptiness.

These combinations are not contradictions; they reflect parallel emotional processes that finally have space to register.

## 2.5 The relationship comes into focus

When ongoing disruption stops, the mind gains capacity to recognise:

- Patterns
- Inconsistencies
- Adaptations made to cope
- The physical and emotional toll.

This awareness can feel confronting, but clarity is a marker of recovery.

## 2.6 Instinct begins to return

As stabilisation progresses, subtle instincts begin re-emerging - the quiet internal cues that were overshadowed by chronic stress.

These may include:

- Recognising what feels appropriate
- Sensing what feels off
- Identifying personal needs
- Noticing what no longer feels tolerable

This is not a "new version" of the self, but a re-emergence of what chronic stress obscured.

There is no single correct way to feel during stabilisation.
No one emerges from prolonged relational stress with everything labelled and neatly filed.
Stabilisation is practical, not polished.

Function is enough for now.

**The Further You Distance Yourself**

The period after leaving a destabilising environment can feel strangely slow. Many people expect immediate answers, full clarity, or a rush of insight. What usually happens, though, is far more methodical. The nervous system recalibrates first. Only then does cognitive clarity begin to return.

Clarity is not a lightning bolt.
It's a gradual re-orientation once the body is no longer busy managing threat.

This chapter explains why clarity often comes later and why this delay is not a flaw, but a predictable part of recovery.

**1. Cognitive Load Reduces Before Insight Appears**

Chronic relational stress forces the brain to prioritise survival functions over reflective thinking. Under prolonged pressure, systems adapt to focus on:

- Minimising conflict
- Tracking mood shifts
- Predicting behaviour
- Suppressing reactions
- Avoiding escalation.

These adaptations are efficient under threat, but costly afterwards.

When the stressor is gone, the brain begins reallocating resources. The prefrontal cortex gradually regains access to functions that were previously unavailable, integrating information, recognising patterns, and making sense of past events (Arnsten, 2009).

This is why clarity often feels delayed.
It wasn't accessible earlier.

## 2. Processing Capacity Changes - Including Micro-Cognition

Chronic relational stress affects more than mood. It impacts subtle, moment-to-moment cognitive functions, often called *micro-cognitions*. These are the small-unit cognitive processes you rely on continuously:

- Organising thoughts
- Shifting attention
- Interpreting tone and context
- Holding short sequences of information
- Making micro-decisions.

Micro-cognition is not a diagnosis. It is a term used in stress and trauma research to describe the fine-grained cognitive operations that are easily disrupted when the nervous system is under sustained strain.

Research shows that chronic stress increases amygdala reactivity and reduces access to the prefrontal cortex, disrupting these smaller executive functions (Arnsten, 2009; Shields et al., 2016).

This is why many people coming out of narcissistic abuse report:

- "I couldn't think straight."
- "I kept second-guessing everything."
- "I couldn't make sense of it until I was out of it."

There is nothing mysterious about this.
Micro-cognition is highly sensitive to stress.
As the system stabilises, these functions gradually return.

### 3. Emotional and Cognitive Systems Come Back Online Out of Sync

Clarity often appears before emotions catch up - or the reverse.

This unevenness is normal.

Research on trauma-affected emotional processing shows that systems recover at different rates (Fisher, 2021). The body may relax before the mind does, or insight may emerge before a person feels ready to engage with it.

### 4. Memory Integration Improves Without Active Effort

Memory under chronic stress becomes fragmented. Not erased, but disorganised.

When the nervous system is no longer bracing, the hippocampus functions more effectively (McEwen & McEwen, 2017). Stored experiences begin linking together in ways that were not possible under pressure.

This is why clarity can feel like:

- Pieces falling into place
- Patterns emerging
- Timelines making sense
- Behaviours that once felt "isolated" suddenly forming a coherent picture.

The system is integrating information that was previously stored in survival mode.

## 5. Recognition Replaces Confusion

Distance removes interference.
This alone creates a significant shift.

Once the environment is stable:

- You can see what was patterned rather than personal
- Behaviour that once felt "unpredictable" becomes recognisable
- You may find language for experiences that previously made no sense.

This isn't overanalysis.
Its cognitive capacity returning.

It's the "what the fuck just happened" moment - when clarity finally lands.

## 6. The Smoke and Mirrors Fall Away

Unpredictability trains the brain to ignore its own instincts in favour of monitoring someone else's behaviour. Once the stimulus is gone, those instincts resume their normal function.

Small things begin to rise to the surface:

- Subtle comments
- Contradictions
- Inconsistencies
- Moments you minimised
- Feelings you dismissed at the time.

This isn't rumination.
It's the nervous system no longer fighting interference.

*Small things float up when the smoke and mirrors are no longer in play — that's when you have capacity for clarity.*

### 7. Clarity Is a Physiological Process

Nothing in this stage requires emotional analysis or cognitive drilling.

Clarity emerges naturally as:

- The threat response decreases
- Micro-cognition improves
- Memory systems link properly
- Instincts regain accuracy
- The prefrontal cortex becomes more available.

Understanding this helps remove any shame around "not seeing it sooner."
You couldn't see it sooner.
Your biology was occupied.

Clarity after distance is not delayed insight.
It is restored function.

### What Recovery Isn't

When people reach the point of distance - whether physical, emotional, or both - there is often an unspoken expectation that recovery should feel clear, uplifting, or purposeful. Many people believe they should immediately feel relief or empowerment. That expectation doesn't come from clinical reality. It comes from the way recovery is portrayed culturally: as something linear, emotional, and transformative.

This chapter clarifies what recovery *is not*, so the reader can understand that their experience doesn't indicate failure, resistance, or "not coping." It indicates a nervous system and cognitive system recalibrating after chronic strain.

## 1. Recovery is not instantaneous clarity

Distance creates the conditions for clarity; it does not provide clarity on demand.
Cognitive processing remains affected by:

- Residual stress activation (Arnsten, 2009)
- Delayed cognitive appraisal (Lazarus & Folkman, 1984)
- Gradual prefrontal cortex recovery after prolonged stress exposure (McEwen & McEwen, 2017).

If you notice inconsistent clarity in the early stages, it reflects normal neurobiological timing. It is not avoidance or ambivalence.

## 2. Recovery is not emotional catharsis

People often expect heightened emotion once they leave the stressful environment.
Instead, many experience:

- Emotional quietness
- Flatness
- Detachment
- Inconsistent feelings.

This is not emotional suppression. It reflects the down-regulation of chronic activation and the body's prioritisation of stabilisation before emotional processing (Fisher, 2021). Emotional systems recalibrate later, not first.

## 3. Recovery is not a "positive mindset" process

Positive thinking does not regulate (though there are always exceptions to this rule):

- Cortisol
- Amygdala hyperreactivity
- Vagal tone
- Disrupted sleep cycles
- GI dysregulation
- Cognitive overload

Evidence shows that physical stabilisation precedes psychological interpretation (Porges, 2011; LeDoux, 2012). Recovery involves biology, not just belief. There's a phrase 'toxic positivity', and there's truth to that. Having been a new-ager myself, there were times when a friend, who was also into the new-age movement, asked me what was it that made me ask for these lessons. I had no contact with that person after that day. Sometimes really shitty things happen to good people, and victim shaming is not helpful.

Please know, I'm not against a positive mindset, in fact, it's part of my goal setting and morning rituals these days, and I think it helped get me through a lot. However, when someone uses it to shame someone that has had a really rough time, I believe it is abhorrent and invalidates their experience, particularly when that person is looking for support.

### 4. Recovery is not linear

People may experience:

- Moments of clarity followed by fog
- Days of steadiness followed by exhaustion
- Fluctuating emotions
- Unexpected memories appearing later rather than sooner.

These variations reflect the oscillation between activation and recovery, not regression. Systems stabilise in waves, not steps.

### 5. Recovery is not immediate self-trust

After prolonged exposure to criticism, inconsistency, or coercive dynamics, self-trust is typically impacted. Research shows disruptions in:

- Executive functioning
- Decision-making confidence
- Fear–safety discrimination
- Microcognition which is the tiny moment-to-moment processes like working memory, attention, and quick decision-making (Sauro & Jorgensen, 2023).

You aren't being "indecisive" You're adapting after long-term vigilance and instability.

## 6. Recovery is not emotional independence

It's common to rely on external validation early in the process. This is not dependency; it reflects the system seeking predictable cues after a period of unpredictability. Regulation often rebuilds through co-regulation with safe people or professionals, before internal regulation is restored.

## 7. Recovery is not an identity shift

A reader may expect to feel like a "new person." Instead, the more accurate process is:

- Recalibration
- Stabilisation
- Reorientation
- Gradual return of instinct
- Slow reconnection with personal preferences and limits.

This is not reinvention, it's restoration.

## 8. Recovery is not quick

Chronic stress affects:

- The HPA axis
- Sleep architecture
- Immune function
- Digestion
- Cognitive clarity
- Emotional processing
- Threat perception.

These systems recover at different speeds. You aren't "taking too long." Be gentle with yourself.

## 9. Recovery is not a moral test

Healing does not require:

- Forgiveness
- Understanding another person's motives
- Emotional closure
- Moral framing
- Reconciling with the past.

## 10. Recovery is not a diagnosis of the other person

Understanding patterns of behaviour does not equate to diagnosing the person who caused harm. The purpose of understanding patterns is:

- To make sense of impact
- To identify what was confusing or destabilising
- To recognise common dynamics
- To reduce self-blame.

It is not about attaching labels or forming conclusions about anyone's mental health.

Recovery doesn't follow the script people expect.
It is quieter, slower, and far more physical than most realise.
Nothing about your timing, feelings, or lack of feelings is

unusual.
This stage isn't meant to be polished.
It's meant to be steady.

## Relearning Your Baseline

When the nervous system finally gets distance from destabilising behaviour, the next stage is not dramatic.
It's quiet.
It's subtle.
And it's mostly physical, long before it becomes emotional.
Relearning your baseline is not about becoming a different person.
It's about recognising the parts of yourself that were overshadowed by chronic stress, constant vigilance, or the need to manage someone else's reactions.

This chapter walks through what this recalibration actually looks like - without pressure, without assumptions, and without any expectation that you should "bounce back." Recovery doesn't work like that.

## 1. Recalibration After Chronic Stress

Chronic interpersonal stress changes how the brain operates. Research shows that prolonged exposure to inconsistency, volatility, or criticism can impair executive functioning, emotional regulation, and micro-cognition. This isn't because someone is "not coping."
It's because the brain was prioritising survival efficiency.

Once the environment becomes safer, that survival mode begins to ease.
Not instantly, gradually.

You may notice shifts like:

- Clearer thinking in short bursts

- Remembering small things again
- Easier decision-making
- Less internal noise
- Fewer moments of over-monitoring your surroundings.

These aren't personality changes.
They are signs that your cognitive load has changed.

## 2. Rediscovering Preferences and Needs

When life has required adapting around someone else's moods, expectations, or demands, your own preferences often get pushed aside.

As stabilisation begins, very ordinary things may resurface:

- What foods you actually enjoy
- How you like your home to feel
- What rest means for you
- How you want to spend your time
- The pace that suits your body.

This isn't self-focus.
It's part of recovery.

Once the brain is no longer spending energy scanning for threat, there's finally space for self-attunement again (McEwen & McEwen, 2017).

It's remarkable how "What do *I* want for dinner?" can feel like a major rediscovery. For me at one stage, it was listening to whatever music I wanted to listen to again.

## 3. Recognising Internal Signals Again

Under prolonged strain, the body changes how it communicates. It quietens some signals and amplifies others to keep you functioning.

As the system steadies, internal cues may become easier to recognise:

- Hunger
- Tiredness
- Interest versus obligation
- Discomfort you don't excuse away
- Preferences that had gone quiet.

This is part of neuroception - the body's pre-conscious safety scanning system (Porges, 2011).
When the sense of threat reduces, more signals make it through.

For many people, this phase feels like "having space in my own head again."

## 4. Choosing Support that Supports You

Not all support stabilises the nervous system. Some responses can quietly retraumatise.

Research on social buffering shows that validating, consistent relationships help reduce physiological stress (Hostinar et al., 2014). The opposite kind - minimising, dismissive, or pressuring - increases it.

Supportive people tend to:

- Take your experience seriously
- Avoid minimising or reframing what happened
- Reject victim-blaming
- Avoid urging reconciliation
- Respect boundaries
- Communicate predictably
- Give space without withdrawing care.

Unhelpful responses often include:

- "You're overreacting."
- "Everyone goes through things like this."
- "Just let it go."
- "Try to fix it with them."

These responses place responsibility back on the person who was harmed.

You deserve support that steadies you, not support that makes you doubt yourself.

**Look for people who validate you, not those that victim-shame you.**

### 5. Why Relational Clarity Takes Time

Clarity about the past often arrives slowly. This delay isn't denial - it's how the brain recovers.

During chronic stress, the prefrontal cortex (the part that tracks patterns and weighs context) is less accessible (Arnsten, 2009). Once pressure reduces, this region becomes more available again.

Over time, you may start noticing:

- Who drains your energy
- Who respects your boundaries
- Who minimises your feelings
- Who listens without rewriting your experience
- Who feels steady
- Who feels familiar in ways that no longer feel healthy.

These insights come from improved cognitive capacity, not emotional "strength."

They come when you have room to think.

### 6. Building Slowly, Not Dramatically

Relearning your baseline doesn't require big declarations or tearing your life apart.
It's the small adjustments that matter:

- Routines that reduce mental load
- Environments that feel predictable
- Commitments that don't stretch you thin
- Communication that is clear and regulated.

This stage is the foundation of deeper recovery. It's steady, slow, and functional.

## Relearning Your Baseline, Part II

Relearning your baseline isn't one moment of clarity, it's a gradual strengthening of internal signals, boundaries, and self-direction. Part I of this book focused on the early physical and emotional settling that happens once the nervous system gains distance from destabilising behaviour. Part II looks at what happens next: the quieter, steadier shifts that gradually restore your sense of self.

This is the stage where life begins to feel less like constant management, and more like something you can participate in again.

## 1. Your Capacity Expands in Small, Measurable Ways

Once the system stabilises, capacity doesn't return as confidence or bold statements.

It returns in increments:

- Conversations that used to drain you now feel easier to navigate
- Your tolerance for chaos decreases (which is a good sign)
- You can recognise red flags earlier
- You pause before reacting
- Your internal "no" becomes clearer

- Expectations feel more realistic.

Research on stress recovery shows that once cognitive load reduces, the prefrontal cortex begins functioning more reliably again (Arnsten, 2009). That's why you may notice you can think more clearly, plan more effectively, or simply follow through with tasks that used to feel overwhelming.

This is not a return to your old self. It's the start of returning to your *actual* self.

## 2. Social Filters Improve

Chronic relational stress distorts how we read people. You may have learned to:

- Minimise your own discomfort
- Over-explain
- Over-accommodate
- Anticipate reactions before they happen
- Ignore internal alarms.

As stabilisation continues, your ability to read social cues becomes more accurate.
Not hypervigilant, appropriate.

Signs this is happening:

- Your patience for poor behaviour lessens
- You recognise inconsistency faster
- You no longer justify patterns that don't feel right
- You prefer steadiness over intensity
- You choose connections based on safety, not familiarity.

This is learning or re-learning discernment.

## 3. Daily Life Becomes Simpler (which is a milestone, not a regression)

When the body and mind recalibrate, daily routines often become surprisingly straightforward. Not boring, but stable.

Examples of this might be:

- Fewer emotional spikes
- Steadier productivity
- Better transitions between tasks
- Lower reactivity to small frustrations
- Fewer moments of internal collapse.

This is supported by evidence showing that improved regulation leads to more efficient executive functioning (McEwen & McEwen, 2017). The absence of chaos helps the system coordinate itself again.

If you find yourself enjoying the luxury of an uneventful week, that's great!

## 4. You Start to Rebuild Your Internal Sense of Safety

Recovery is not only external.
It involves reconstructing your own internal sense of safety - the feeling that your thoughts, instincts, and perceptions are valid.

This strengthening is subtle:

- You check your phone less
- You no longer brace before giving an opinion
- You can disagree calmly
- You're less afraid of being misunderstood
- You trust yourself more than external noise.

It's what happens when neuroception shifts from "threat-dominant" to "safety-dominant" (Porges, 2011).

Your system learns that: *You are allowed to exist without being interrupted, corrected, or destabilised.*

## 5. If You Are Not Able to Leave Your Situation Yet

Not everyone can leave a destabilising or abusive environment immediately - or at all - due to cultural, familial, financial, legal, or safety constraints.

If any of those circumstances apply to you:

**Please seek a trauma-informed therapist or clinician who specialises in narcissistic abuse recovery.**

The information contained in this book cannot replace specialised support, nor can it guide you through high-risk or constrained situations.

A qualified clinician can help you:

- Build internal safety
- Establish micro-boundaries
- Navigate practical obstacles
- Develop strategies for minimising harm
- Maintain psychological clarity in destabilising dynamics.

## 6. Steady Doesn't Mean Finished

Relearning your baseline isn't the final stage of recovery - it's the platform that everything else is built on. What comes next is deeper work: rebuilding identity, reconnecting with meaning, strengthening relational boundaries, and restoring physiological balance.

You're not expected to rush into those stages. This phase is about giving your system the space it needed all along.

## The First Signs of Reconnection

Reconnection doesn't arrive with fireworks, revelations, or a sudden rush of enthusiasm. It shows up quietly, in small increments, often when you're not looking for it. If stabilisation is the phase where the system stops bracing, reconnection is the stage where it starts reaching.

Nothing dramatic.
No forced epiphanies.
Just subtle shifts that tell you your system has enough bandwidth to look outward again.

Below is what reconnection *actually* looks like, based on research, nervous system science, and the lived recovery patterns seen repeatedly in trauma-informed practice.

### 1. Curiosity Returns in Small, Manageable Pieces

After prolonged relational stress, curiosity is one of the first indicators that the nervous system is re-opening.
Not excitement. Not motivation.
Curiosity.

It can look like:

- A mild interest in learning something new
- Reading a paragraph without losing track
- Noticing you want to actually understand something, instead of just getting through the day.

This is consistent with improvements in prefrontal cortical engagement once threat activation decreases (Arnsten, 2009; Fisher, 2021).

It doesn't mean you're "back."
It means your mind is poking its head above the parapet.

## 2. Your Internal Pace Evens Out

When you've lived in survival mode, everything feels urgent, even when nothing is happening.
Reconnection brings small changes in pace:

- Fewer adrenaline-driven decisions
- The ability to pause without fear
- Less internal rushing
- Noticing you can complete a task without bracing.

This reflects the gradual recalibration of autonomic states as parasympathetic regulation improves (Porges, 2011).

## 3. Preferences Start Returning

During prolonged stress, the system doesn't prioritise preference, it prioritises survival.
Reconnection signals that the brain now has room for choice again.

You might notice:

- A food you actually feel like eating
- A colour you gravitate toward
- A TV show you genuinely want to watch
- A decision you make without fear of repercussions.

This isn't indulgence; it's the re-emergence of your identity underneath chronic activation.

## 4. Your Capacity for Connection With Others Changes

This phase is not about entering new relationships or forcing social reconnection.
It's about noticing small internal markers that your system is less defended.

These markers can include:

- Tolerating longer conversations
- Enjoying brief interactions
- Feeling safe enough to maintain eye contact
- Recognising when someone is kind without suspicion
- Seeking gentle company instead of isolation.

Interpersonal neurobiology research shows that once hypervigilance decreases, social engagement systems begin to re-activate (Porges, 2011).

It's not a push toward people, more so it's the absence of needing to keep everyone at arm's length.

## 5. Your Sense of Humour Shifts

Humour changes meaningfully once the nervous system has space.
This is often one of the most recognisable signs of reconnection.

Not performative humour.
Not humour used as defence.
Just a small, genuine spark of amusement.

A slight chuckle at something trivial.
The capacity to find something mildly ridiculous without collapsing into cynicism.

It's another physiological sign that the threat response is diminishing.

## 6. You Notice Small Threads of Future Thinking

Future thinking isn't planning a new life.
It's the internal permission to think beyond the next 12 hours.

It might appear as:

- Wondering what you'd like to learn
- Considering a change without panic
- Imagining a small improvement in your daily life
- Thinking in "maybe" instead of "never".

This corresponds with improved prefrontal cortical functioning and reduced limbic dominance (LeDoux, 2012).

Future thinking is not pressure - it's possibility.

## 7. Your Body Begins to Trust You Again

Reconnection includes the physical experience of noticing your body as part of you again, not just a vehicle for survival.

You may feel:

- Hunger cues returning
- A desire to stretch or move
- Easier breathing
- Fewer stress-related physical symptoms
- The ability to sit still without adrenaline kicking in.

The system re-associates the body with safety rather than threat, which is a critical shift in trauma recovery (Fisher, 2021).

## 8. You Begin to Look at Your Story Without Overwhelm

This is not about deep emotional processing, nor is it an invitation to revisit anything traumatic. It's the simple ability to acknowledge what you lived through, with steadier footing.

You may think:

"That wasn't okay."

"That was harder than I realised."

"I understand what was happening now."

There is no emotional assignment in this. Just increased coherence - the ability to hold a memory without your system flooding.

It's cognitive processing returning to stability (Hinojosa et al., 2017).

# PART III

# CHAPTER FOURTEEN

# The Hogan Method: What it is and isn't

People often reach this part of the book expecting a "how-to" list, a shortcut, or a formula they can apply in a weekend and call it done. Recovery from narcissistic abuse does not work like that. The Hogan Method wasn't created to give you steps to rush through, or a checklist to "fix" yourself. It exists because after decades in clinical practice, teaching, research and lived experience, it became clear that most people needed something they weren't getting anywhere else: a grounded physiological framework to help the body stabilise after prolonged relational stress.

This method is *not* therapy.
It is *not* a substitute for trauma-informed psychological care.
It does *not* diagnose, treat, or cure anything.
It is not built on spiritual philosophy, pop psychology, or wishful thinking.

It is built on a simple premise that stands the test of research and clinical experience:

**Your body doesn't lie.**
And when it has lived in threat long enough, it needs support to find its footing again.

The Hogan Method works alongside therapy, not instead of it. It is a stabilising framework - body first, clarity second. Most survivors try to do the opposite: they push themselves to "understand everything" while their physiology is still in survival mode. That is like trying to rebuild a house while the fire is still burning. This method helps you lower the flames so you can see what you're working with.

## 1. Why This Method Exists

Prolonged exposure to inconsistent, manipulative, or controlling behaviour has measurable effects on the body. This isn't dramatic language, it's physiology. Chronic interpersonal stress alters the nervous system, disrupts sleep, undermines digestion, erodes energy reserves, and blunts executive functioning (Arnsten, 2009; Porges, 2011; McEwen & McEwen, 2017). Many people coming out of narcissistic environments don't realise they've been living in a threat-adapted body.

Talk therapy often focuses on story, meaning, and emotional processing.
Those are important.
But your body needs a foundation first.

Without it, people often feel:

- Foggy
- Overwhelmed
- Unable to make decisions
- Emotionally flat
- Constantly on edge
- Inconsistent in their reactions.

These aren't personality traits. They're physiological responses to chronic stress.

The Hogan Method addresses this by focusing on stabilisation before interpretation.

## 2. What the Method *Is*

A structured, body-first framework grounded in:

- Stress physiology
- Nervous system regulation
- Naturopathic principles
- Nutritional biochemistry
- Herbal support (evidence-based, not prescriptive)
- Clinical observation across decades of practice
- Lived understanding of relational trauma.

It gives you clarity, not conclusions.
It gives you structure, not diagnosis.
It gives you understanding, not pressure.

This method recognises that the ability to reflect, plan, and reconnect is only possible once the stress physiology has space to recalibrate. In other words:

**You need a stable platform within your body while you are rebuilding.**

## 3. What the Method *Isn't*

This is not a program that promises transformation in a timeline.
It is not a replacement for trauma-informed therapy or medical care.
It is not a spiritual bypass.
It does not blame, shame, or pathologise you.
It does not frame survival adaptations as "problems."
It does not encourage reprocessing of traumatic memories.
It is not about pushing yourself harder - quite the opposite.

There are no reparenting scripts, no "visualise your healed self" tasks.
Nothing here is performative.

Everything here is physiological, practical, stabilising, and achievable.

### 4. Why Body Recovery Matters

Your mind cannot settle until your biology does. That's not opinion; it's how the stress response works.

Chronic relational stress triggers:

- Heightened amygdala activation (LeDoux, 2012)
- Suppressed prefrontal functioning (Arnsten, 2009)
- Dysregulated vagal tone (Porges, 2011)
- Elevated allostatic load (McEwen & McEwen, 2017).

When those systems are running in the background, clarity becomes inconsistent and emotional responses can feel unpredictable. Trying to "think your way out" of this is like trying to reason with adrenaline.

The Hogan Method focuses on helping the system step out of chronic activation, so that clarity can return naturally. Once the body is no longer spending all its resources on survival, there is finally room for self-reflection, calm, and choice.

### 5. What You Can Expect From This Section

In the chapters ahead, you'll learn:

- How chronic relational stress affects the body
- Why your symptoms made sense
- The physiological order in which recovery tends to unfold
- How the body signals stabilisation
- What early signs of reconnection look like
- How sleep, digestion, and energy shift during recovery
- Which nutrient systems are commonly impacted by prolonged stress

- How herbal and nutritional support can assist stabilisation (not treat trauma)
- What "listening to your body" means -without the fluff.

Nothing in this section will ask you to interpret your trauma. Nothing here will ask you to revisit memories. Nothing will assume anything about your emotional landscape. This is the calm, grounded, stabilising part of the book.

## 6. A Note Before We Begin

If you've spent years doubting yourself, overriding your instincts, or apologising for your own exhaustion, the next chapters may feel strangely practical. That's deliberate. People underestimate how physical this recovery is. Understanding the body isn't the whole journey, but it's a good start.

You don't need to fix everything right now. You just need your system to stop sprinting inside its own skin.

The work ahead is steady, clear, grounded, and entirely possible.

## Early Physical Changes in Stabilisation

When the body is no longer dealing with constant relational stress, the earliest shifts are physical. These changes are often subtle, practical and based entirely on physiology. They're not "recovery"; they're the body reallocating resources that were previously diverted into managing threat.

This chapter outlines what you might experience as the first physical signs that your system is adjusting to increased safety.

## 1. Breathing Becomes Less Shallow

Chronic interpersonal stress activates the sympathetic nervous system and reduces diaphragmatic movement. Research shows that prolonged threat cues increase shallow, upper-chest breathing (Boiten, 1998) and reduce autonomic flexibility (Thayer & Lane, 2000).

As the environment becomes safer:

- Breathing deepens
- Shoulders drop
- Chest tightness reduces
- Sighing increases (a vagal recovery cue).

These shifts are not psychological.
They indicate a reduction in sustained sympathetic arousal.

## 2. Muscle Tension Begins to Ease

Muscles carry a significant portion of stress physiology. Extended activation of the hypothalamic-pituitary-adrenal (HPA) axis increases muscle tension and reduces recovery capacity (McEwen & McEwen, 2017).

You may notice:

- Jaw unclenching
- Reduced neck and shoulder tightness
- Fewer tension headaches
- Less bracing during rest.

This isn't relaxation.
It's the body standing down from baseline defence.

### 3. Energy Levels Begin to Stabilise

Cortisol dysregulation often leads to fatigue, irritability, and unpredictable energy spikes (Gianaros & Wager, 2015). When the stressor is removed:

- Morning energy may return
- Afternoon crashes may lessen
- Jitteriness may reduce
- Exhaustion may become more predictable, rather than overwhelming.

This isn't "feeling energised."
It's reduced metabolic over-compensation.

### 4. Digestive Function starts to settle

Chronic stress suppresses digestive activity through sympathetic dominance, affecting motility, secretion and gut–brain signalling (Mayer, 2011).

With distance from the stressor:

- Appetite stabilises
- Nausea becomes less frequent
- Bloating and cramping ease
- Bowel patterns normalise.

These shifts happen because vagal function improves - not because someone is "thinking positively."

### 5. Sleep Begins to Shift

Sleep often changes early, but not evenly. Stress hormones influence circadian rhythm, dream intensity and sleep depth (van der Helm & Walker, 2009).

Common early-phase patterns include:

- Deeper sleep in short segments
- Occasional oversleeping
- Difficulty falling asleep, despite tiredness
- Periods of fragmented sleep
- Vivid dreams or stress-processing dreams.

All of these reflect the nervous system beginning to recalibrate.

## 6. The Immune System Responds More Appropriately

The immune system is strongly affected by chronic relational stress. Long-term activation elevates inflammatory markers and suppresses certain immune responses (Segerstrom & Miller, 2004; Dhabhar, 2014).

Once the stressor is removed:

- Minor infections may reduce
- Inflammation-related symptoms may ease
- Skin conditions may improve
- Recovery from simple illnesses becomes easier.

However, and this is the key point, the immune system generally stabilises later than the nervous system or digestion. Research shows:

- Immune recovery follows the reduction of cortisol and catecholamines
- Inflammatory pathways require more time to downregulate
- The immune system may lag behind other systems by weeks or months.

References: Segerstrom & Miller, 2004; McEwen & McEwen, 2017; Dhabhar, 2014.

Early changes do occur, but full immune recovery tends to be a later-stage outcome.

## 7. Headaches, Migraines and Sensory Sensitivity Can Improve

Stress can heighten pain sensitivity, increase muscular tension, and alter sensory thresholds (Bushnell et al., 2013).

You may notice:

- Fewer headaches
- Reduced sound/light sensitivity
- Less jaw pain
- Fewer tension-triggered migraines.

These changes reflect reduced autonomic load.

## When Cognitive Function Begins to Return

As stabilisation progresses, the next noticeable shift is cognitive. Not dramatic clarity, not sudden insight, but the slow return of basic mental functions that were compromised under chronic relational stress.

This chapter outlines what commonly returns first and why, without implying that the process is linear or identical for everyone.

## 1. Executive Functioning Improves in Small, Practical Ways

Chronic relational stress affects the prefrontal cortex, reducing access to planning, decision-making, task-sequencing and working memory (Arnsten, 2009). When excessive activation reduces, these functions begin to come back online - often quietly.

You may notice:

- Tasks feeling less overwhelming
- Better ability to plan small steps
- Improved follow-through
- Reduced procrastination from cognitive fatigue.

These improvements are not "motivation." They reflect increased prefrontal accessibility once the system is no longer dominated by threat-response circuits.

## 2. Micro-Cognition Starts to Stabilise

Micro-cognition refers to the small cognitive actions that support daily functioning - organising thoughts, shifting attention, retrieving words, sequencing steps and processing information efficiently.

Under chronic relational stress, micro-cognition can become impaired because attentional and memory resources are continually redirected toward monitoring safety (Fisher, 2021; LeDoux, 2012).

When the stressor is no longer present:

- Word-finding becomes easier
- Task-switching is less draining
- Mental organisation increases
- Simple problem-solving improves.

These changes reflect reduced competing demands on cognitive load.

## 3. The Capacity for Perspective-Taking Expands

Chronic stress constricts cognitive flexibility, making it difficult to consider alternatives, reframe situations or evaluate things without urgency (McEwen & McEwen, 2017).

With stabilisation:

- The need for immediate conclusions reduces
- The ability to think in broader terms returns
- Interpretation becomes more balanced
- Black-and-white thinking eases.

This is not "becoming positive." It is cognitive bandwidth widening.

## 4. Emotional Reasoning and Catastrophising Reduce

Stress heightens threat perception, increasing tendencies toward worst-case scenario thinking (LeDoux & Pine, 2016).

As stabilisation progresses:

- Emotional reasoning becomes less dominant
- Catastrophic expectations lessen
- Interpretation becomes more aligned with context
- The internal "alarm" is not constantly firing.

These changes occur because the limbic system is less activated, not because someone is "trying harder."

## 5. Attention Capacity Improves

Attention is heavily influenced by threat-response systems. When the nervous system is bracing, attention becomes narrow, rigid or scattered (Arnsten, 2009).

With recovery:

- Focus increases in short bursts

- Attention switching becomes more effortless
- Sustained attention slowly returns
- Tasks requiring concentration feel more manageable.

Readers often mistake this for "finally getting it together." It's physiology, not personality.

## 6. The Ability to Make Decisions Reappears

Decision paralysis is common during and after prolonged stress, because executive areas are compromised, and the system prioritises safety scanning over decision processing (Porges, 2011).

With stabilisation:

- Minor decisions feel less overwhelming
- Choices don't feel dangerous
- The internal sense of "what's okay" becomes clearer
- The need to consult others reduces.

This is one of the most encouraging early cognitive shifts - and also one of the most subtle.

## 7. Retrospective Clarity Increases

This is not rumination.
It is simply the brain reviewing information that was previously drowned out by stress physiology.

As cognitive load decreases:

- Past events can be evaluated with more accuracy
- Patterns may become more visible
- Inconsistencies in previous dynamics make more sense
- Self-blame reduces because processing becomes more grounded.

This is not a psychological breakthrough.
It's cognitive availability.

## 8. High-Functioning Survival and What Changes During Recalibration

Not everyone collapses outwardly during prolonged stress. Many people continue functioning at a high level - at work, at home, academically, socially - even while their internal systems are under significant strain. Research shows that high-functioning under chronic stress is maintained through overactivation of compensatory neural networks, increased cortisol availability, and habit-driven behaviour patterns that can mask the underlying load (McEwen & McEwen, 2017; Fisher, 2021).

This form of functioning often relies on:

- Structure
- Responsibility
- Habit
- Hypervigilance
- Adrenaline-supported productivity.

When stabilisation begins, these compensatory systems don't immediately know they can stand down. People who have functioned at a high level for years may feel more disoriented by the return of cognitive capacity than people whose external functioning declined.

Common shifts include:

- Mental fatigue appearing once the "emergency mode" drops
- Temporary decreases in productivity
- Noticing how many tasks were previously completed on autopilot
- The sense of "coming down" from internal overdrive
- The reappearance of needs that were previously ignored.

These are not failures.
They are signs that the nervous system is no longer overriding itself to meet expectations.

### Example - A Woman Balancing Work and Young Children

A woman in a demanding role with young children may not notice the cognitive toll of prolonged relational stress, until the system finally has room to adjust. During the stressful period, she may have:

- Maintained routines without pause
- Handled school drop-offs, lunches, bedtime, work meetings
- Run on efficiency rather than presence
- Responded quickly to every need because slowing down didn't feel safe.

Once stabilisation begins, she may start to notice:

- Struggling to multitask in the same way
- Pockets of exhaustion she previously pushed through
- Emotional signals she had no capacity to register
- Irritability that isn't about her children, but about depleted reserves
- Forgetfulness as the brain shifts out of survival efficiency.

She might find herself sitting down for a moment and realising she hasn't stopped all day. Or noticing she can finally take a slow breath once the house is quiet. Or recognising that she feels a little clearer at times, not in every moment or dramatically, but in ways that were previously unavailable.

These are signs of recalibration, not decline. Her functioning hasn't disappeared, it's simply becoming less adrenaline-dependent and more sustainable.

## 8. Why High-Functioning People Often Experience Delayed Cognitive Return

People who maintain high-functioning roles under stress tend to rely heavily on procedural memory and habit loops. Research shows that under stress, the brain shifts from flexible, prefrontal-based functioning toward more rigid habit-based networks (Arnsten, 2009). When stabilisation begins, the transition back toward cognitive flexibility can feel disjointed.

Common temporary experiences include:

- "Why am I suddenly tired all the time?"
  (Because the body is no longer suppressing fatigue.)
- "Why can't I make simple decisions?"
  (Because micro-cognition is rebalancing.)
- "Why do I feel off when nothing is wrong?"
  (Because the absence of stress feels unfamiliar.)

These shifts reflect recovery, not regression.

## 9. A Note on Expectations

You might expect cognitive recovery to feel dramatic - as if clarity should arrive in a single moment. In reality, it tends to show up in small, practical ways first, including finding your keys more easily, remembering why you walked into the room or finishing a task, without stopping five times. These are the real indicators of cognitive stabilisation.

# CHAPTER FIFTEEN

# The Naturopathic Bridge

When you reach the point where the chaos has stopped and your system finally has room to breathe, a different kind of work begins. The psychological fog starts to lift in small pockets, but the physical body is often still catching up.

For many people, this is the stage where the question becomes: **"What can I do to support myself now?"**

This is where a naturopathic perspective fits in. Not as a cure, not as a shortcut, and not as a replacement for trauma-informed therapy, but as the part that **helps your body stabilise so you can do the rest of the work with more capacity**.

The Hogan Method brings these pieces together in a structured, practical way. It looks at:

- What prolonged relational stress has done to your biology
- Which systems are still running on old survival settings
- What nutrients may have been depleted
- How digestion, sleep, hormones, and immunity have been affected
- How your nervous system is recalibrating
- What supports may help your body return to equilibrium.

This isn't about fixing symptoms individually. It's about understanding that each part of the body responds to stress in predictable ways - and each part needs something slightly different to come back online.

Most people don't realise how physical the fallout can be. You might notice:

- Energy fluctuations
- Disrupted sleep
- Digestive discomfort
- Muscle tension
- Lowered immunity
- Difficulty concentrating
- Irritability
- Feeling "wired and tired"
- A sense of being emotionally flat
- Not feeling like yourself at all
- Pain and inflammation.

These aren't personal weaknesses.
They're biological responses to prolonged pressure.

Naturopathic support simply gives the body what it needs so it can stabilise, repair, and regain balance. It's not dramatic or mysterious - it's physiology, gently supported.

The Hogan Method draws on:

- Clinical nutrition
- Herbal medicine
- Mind–body support
- Sleep and circadian repair
- Digestive recovery
- Nervous system regulation
- Simple behavioural shifts.

Every person's situation is unique, and no two bodies respond to stress in the same way. That's why the approach is tailored.

You've spent the last chapters understanding **why** your system reacted the way it did - why confusion occurs, why the body adapts, and why the aftermath feels the way it does.

Now we move into **what may help**, starting with the physical foundations.

This next chapter focuses on the first layer of that support: **nutrients that may help the body stabilise during the early and middle stages of recovery.**

Herbal medicines will follow.
Then adjunct therapies.
Then lifestyle supports that form part of a steady return to equilibrium.

None of this replaces therapy or emotional support. But giving the body what it needs reduces strain, improves capacity, and provides a solid base from which psychological healing becomes more manageable.

When your biology begins functioning more efficiently, everything else becomes easier to carry. This is the stage where physical steadiness starts to support emotional steadiness - and that's where we go next.

**15.1 - Nervous System Nutrients**

Chronic stress places the nervous system under continuous demand. Over time, this can deplete key nutrients that keep the system stable, regulate nerve signalling, support cognition, and maintain emotional steadiness. The nutrients in this chapter are not "quick fixes." They're foundational ingredients your brain and nervous system rely on to function.

When people experience prolonged stress, burnout, or the physiological effects of narcissistic abuse, it is common to see patterns of depletion across these nutrients. The goal here is not diagnosis - it's clarity. When you understand how nutrients interact with stress physiology, you can make informed decisions about support. However, always consult your qualified health care professional to determine if there's an underlying

## Magnesium

### 1. What it does

Magnesium supports over 300 biochemical processes, many of them directly involved in nervous system regulation. It helps keep nerve signalling stable, supports neurotransmitter balance, and prevents excessive excitatory activity (Groenendijk et al., 2021).

### 2. How stress affects it

Chronic stress increases magnesium loss through the kidneys (Kirkland et al., 2018).
This means the more stressed someone is, the faster magnesium is depleted.

### 3. Symptoms of low levels

Evidence-supported symptoms include:

- Muscle tension
- Eye twitches
- Restlessness
- Increased startle response
- Headaches
- Irritability
- Light-sleeping or waking unrefreshed.

### 4. Why it matters in stress recovery

When magnesium levels are low, the nervous system becomes more reactive. Restoring levels often supports calmer sleep, more stable moods, and reduced physical tension.

### 5. Food sources

Leafy greens, nuts, seeds, legumes, whole grains.

### 6. When supplementation may help

Useful when symptoms of tension, poor sleep quality, or excessive nervous system activation are present - ideally under guidance from a qualified practitioner.

### References

Groenendijk, I. et al. (2021)...

Kirkland, A. et al., (2018)...

(Full reference list will appear at the end of Part 3.)

## Thiamine (Vitamin B1)

### 1. What it does

Thiamine supports nerve conduction, glucose metabolism in the brain, and stress resilience (Michels et al., 2021).

### 2. How stress affects it

Stress increases metabolic demand. Because thiamine is required for energy production in nerve cells, chronic activation can deplete it faster.

### 3. Symptoms of low levels

- Fatigue
- Brain fog
- Irritability
- Difficulty concentrating

- Neuropathy-like tingling (when significantly low).

### 4. Why it matters in stress recovery

Thiamine helps restore normal cognitive processing and energy production in the brain.

### 5. Food sources

Whole grains, sunflower seeds, legumes, lean meats.

### 6. When supplementation may help

When mental fatigue or cognitive slowing is prominent.

## Riboflavin (VitaminB2)

### 1. What it does

Riboflavin helps convert food into usable energy and supports myelin (nerve insulation) and mitochondrial stability.

### 2. How stress affects it

Stress increases oxidative load, which uses more riboflavin for antioxidant enzymes (Powers, 2020).

### 3. Symptoms of low levels

- Low energy
- Light sensitivity
- Cracks at the corners of the mouth
- Migraines in some cases (supported by evidence).

### 4. Why it matters in stress recovery

Helps stabilise energy and supports neurological function.

### 5. Food sources

Eggs, dairy, almonds, mushrooms.

### 6. When supplementation may help

When energy-related symptoms or migraine patterns are present.

## Niacin (Vitamin B3)

### 1. What it does

Niacin is essential for cellular energy, nervous system stability, and neurotransmitter synthesis.

### 2. How stress affects it

Chronic stress increases turnover of NAD/NADP, which depend on niacin.

### 3. Symptoms of low levels

- Fatigue
- Low mood
- Poor concentration
- Skin flushing/sensitivity (if very depleted).

### 4. Why it matters in stress recovery

Supports cognitive steadiness and restores cellular energy.

### 5. Food sources

Poultry, fish, whole grains, peanuts.

## Pantothenic Acid (Vitamin B5)

### 1. What it does

B5 supports adrenal hormone synthesis and is essential for forming acetylcholine, an important neurotransmitter for attention and memory.

### 2. How stress affects it

Sustained stress increases adrenal hormone production, which uses more B5.

### 3. Symptoms of low levels

- Profound fatigue
- Difficulty coping with stress
- Irritability
- Sleep disturbances.

### 4. Why it matters in stress recovery

Helps balance the stress response and supports energy.

### 5. Food sources

Avocado, chicken, whole grains, lentils.

## Pyridoxine (Vitamin B6)

### 1. What it does

B6 is required to produce GABA, serotonin, dopamine, and melatonin - the neurotransmitters most impacted by stress (Parletta et al., 2016).

### 2. How stress affects it

Stress and inflammation increase B6 utilisation.

### 3. Symptoms of low levels

- Anxiety or agitation
- Low mood
- Sleep issues
- PMS symptoms (in some individuals).

### 4. Why it matters in stress recovery

Improves neurotransmitter balance, which can support mood regulation and sleep.

### 5. Food sources

Bananas, poultry, chickpeas, potatoes.

## Folate (Vitamin B9)

### 1. What it does

Folate supports methylation, neurotransmitter formation, and cognitive processing.

### 2. How stress affects it

Chronic stress and inflammation can impair folate pathways (Morris et al., 2020).

### 3. Symptoms of low levels

- Low mood
- Cognitive fog
- Fatigue

- Reduced stress tolerance.

**4. Why it matters in recovery**

Supports mental clarity and emotional steadiness.

**5. Food sources**

Leafy greens, legumes, citrus.

**Methylfolate**

**1. What it does**

The active form of folate used directly for neurotransmitter production.

**2. Why stress affects it**

If methylation is impaired or folate intake is low, stress resilience decreases.

**3. Symptoms of low availability**

Similar to folate but may present with stronger cognitive symptoms.

**4. Notes**

Not everyone needs methylfolate - this is where practitioner support is essential.

### Cobalamin (Vitamin B12)

**1. What it does**

Essential for nerve insulation (myelin), energy production, and mood regulation, blood cell formation

**2. How stress affects it**

Stress may reduce absorption in some individuals due to GI disruption.

**3. Symptoms of low levels**

- Pins and needles
- Low mood
- Fatigue
- Memory lapses
- "Brain fog".

**4. Why it matters in recovery**

Supports the nervous system's ability to return to baseline.

**5. Food sources**

Animal products, fortified foods.

### Choline

**1. What it does**

Choline helps form acetylcholine, which is essential for memory, attention, and nervous system communication.

**2. How stress affects it**

More choline is used during high cortisol states.

### 3. Symptoms of low levels

- Memory issues
- Poor concentration
- Fatigue
- Mood changes.

### 4. Why it matters in recovery

Supports cognitive function and stabilises neural communication.

### 5. Food sources

Eggs, soy, legumes, fish.

## Inositol

### 1. What it does

Acts as a signalling molecule in the brain. Supports serotonin, insulin regulation, and stress reactivity.

### 2. How stress affects it

Stress alters neurotransmitter pathways that inositol supports.

### 3. Symptoms of low levels

- Anxiety
- Mood imbalance
- Sleep disturbance
- Sugar cravings (insulin-related).

### 4. Why it matters in recovery

Helps restore balance in stress-affected neural pathways.

### 5. Food sources

Fruits, beans, grains, nuts.

## 15.2 - Energy Nutrients

When someone has lived with long-term stress, the body pulls nutrients toward survival priorities - keeping you alert, keeping you upright, and keeping you going. Energy production is one of the first areas affected, and it's one of the most noticeable areas to improve when the right supports are in place. This chapter looks at nutrients that directly support the body's energy pathways, why stress depletes them, and what symptoms someone might notice when levels are low.

### 1. B Vitamins - The Core Energy Group

The B vitamins act as co-factors in almost every energy-producing pathway in the body. When stress is prolonged, the demand for these nutrients increases, and levels can drop. Replenishing them can support steadier energy, clearer thinking, and recovery from fatigue.

#### 1.1 Vitamin B1 (Thiamine)

**What it does in the body**

Thiamine plays a central role in converting carbohydrates into usable energy. It's required for nerve conduction, muscle function, and the biochemical processes that keep the brain fuelled throughout the day.

**How stress impacts it**

Prolonged stress increases metabolic demand, which increases the body's utilisation of thiamine. Over time, this can contribute to functional depletion.

## Symptoms of low thiamine

Evidence shows deficiency can present as:

- Persistent fatigue
- Irritability
- Low mood
- Cognitive fog
- Muscle weakness
- Reduced exercise tolerance.

## Why it matters in recovery.

When thiamine is insufficient, energy pathways slow down, and even basic daily activities can feel harder.

## Food sources

Whole grains, legumes, nuts, seeds, pork, fortified cereals.

## When supplementation may help

Useful when energy is consistently low, especially after prolonged stress or poor dietary intake.

## 1.2 Vitamin B2 (Riboflavin)

### What it does

Riboflavin is essential for mitochondrial energy production and helps convert other B vitamins into their active forms.

### Stress impact

Increased energy demand during stress accelerates riboflavin utilisation.

### Symptoms of low riboflavin

- Fatigue
- Sore or burning eyes
- Cracked lips or corners of the mouth
- Light sensitivity
- Headaches.

### Why it matters.

Low riboflavin impairs the cellular processes that generate ATP (cellular energy).

### Food sources

Dairy, eggs, lean meats, almonds, mushrooms, leafy greens.

### 1.3 Vitamin B3 (Niacin)

### What it does

Niacin is involved in more than 400 enzyme reactions, many of which relate directly to energy production and nervous system health.

### Stress impact

Chronic stress can increase the body's need for niacin due to heightened metabolic activity.

### Symptoms of low Niacin

- Persistent tiredness
- Irritability
- Poor stress tolerance
- Concentration problems
- Skin flushing or sensitivity.

**Why it matters.**

Adequate Niacin supports stable mood and clearer thinking during recovery.

**Food sources**

Poultry, fish, beef, peanuts, whole grains.

### 1.4 Vitamin B5 (Pantothenic Acid)

**What it does**

Pantothenic acid supports adrenal gland function and helps synthesise coenzyme A, which is essential for energy production.

**Stress impact**

Stress increases adrenal activity, which increases demand for vitamin B5.

**Symptoms of low pantothenic acid**

- Fatigue
- Headaches
- Sleep disturbances
- Muscle cramps
- Irritability.

**Why it matters.**

Low B5 can contribute to "wired and tired" feelings during prolonged stress.

**Food sources**

Eggs, poultry, whole grains, avocados, legumes.

### 1.5 Vitamin B6 (Pyridoxine)

**What it does**

B6 is required for neurotransmitter synthesis (serotonin, dopamine, GABA) and supports energy and nervous system stability.

**Stress impact**

Chronic stress draws heavily on B6 because of its role in neurotransmitter regulation.

**Symptoms of low B6**

- Irritability
- Low mood
- Poor stress tolerance
- Brain fog
- Premenstrual mood changes
- Tingling or numbness.

**Why it matters.**

Adequate B6 supports mental clarity, stable mood, and resilience during recovery.

**Food sources**

Poultry, fish, bananas, chickpeas, potatoes.

### 1.6 Vitamin B12 (Cobalamin)

**What it does**

B12 is essential for red blood cell formation, nerve function, and DNA synthesis.

**Stress impact**

Chronic stress may reduce absorption and increase utilisation.

**Symptoms of low B12**

- Extreme fatigue
- Breathlessness
- Pallor
- Memory issues
- Tingling in hands or feet
- Low mood or irritability.

**Why it matters.**

B12 deficiency significantly impacts energy levels and cognitive function.

**Food sources**

Animal products, such as eggs, meat, dairy, fish. Vegetarians/vegans often require supplementation.

## 1.7 Folate (Vitamin B9)

**What it does**

Folate is essential for methylation, neurotransmitter production, and energy metabolism.

**Stress impact**

Stress can impair folate absorption and increase demand.

**Symptoms of low folate**

- Low energy
- Difficulty concentrating

- Low mood
- Irritability
- Mouth ulcers.

**Why it matters.**

Low folate can contribute to fatigue and decreased resilience.

**Food sources**

Leafy greens, legumes, citrus, beets, fortified grains.

## 1.8 Iron

**What it does**

Iron is essential for transporting oxygen around the body. Without adequate oxygen supply, energy drops quickly.

**Stress impact**

Chronic stress can affect iron absorption and storage.

**Symptoms of low iron**

- Exhaustion
- Breathlessness
- Dizziness
- Pale skin
- Hair loss
- Brittle nails
- Headaches.

**Why it matters.**

Iron deficiency can significantly worsen fatigue and concentration issues.

## Food sources

Red meat, poultry, legumes, spinach, fortified cereals.

## 2. Additional Energy-Supporting Nutrients

### 2.1 Magnesium

Although also a nervous system nutrient, magnesium contributes directly to ATP production - the body's primary energy currency.

### Symptoms of low magnesium

- Fatigue
- Muscle cramps
- Headaches
- Eye twitches
- Poor stress tolerance.

### 2.2 Iodine

### What it does

Supports thyroid hormone production - a key regulator of metabolic energy.

### Symptoms of low iodine

- Fatigue
- Weight changes
- Dry skin
- Feeling cold
- Cognitive slowing.

## 2.3 Selenium

### What it does

Supports thyroid hormone activation and antioxidant defence.

### Symptoms of low Selenium

- Low mood
- Sluggishness
- Poor immunity
- Muscle weakness.

## 2.4 Chromium

### What it does

Helps stabilise blood sugar levels, preventing energy crashes.

### Symptoms of low chromium

- Fatigue after meals
- Sugar cravings
- Brain fog
- Irritability.

## 2.5 Inositol

### What it does

Supports cellular communication and energy balance in the brain.

### Symptoms of low inositol

Not a classical deficiency, but low intake is associated with:

- Poor stress tolerance
- Anxiousness
- Disrupted energy patterns.

## 15.3 — Sleep Support Nutrients

Sleep is usually one of the first things affected when you live with long-term stress. Under chronic activation, the body prioritises survival systems, not rest. Once the pressure reduces, the physiology that supports sleep begins to recalibrate, and certain micronutrients have strong evidence for helping this process along.

These nutrients do not "fix" insomnia on their own. They support the biochemical pathways involved in settling the nervous system, regulating sleep architecture, and improving sleep quality - particularly, when the body has been under strain for a prolonged period.

Each nutrient below is included because there is **credible, peer-reviewed evidence** linking it with sleep or sleep-related physiological functions. Always consult your qualified health care professional to determine if there's an underlying physiological condition that also needs attention.

### 1. Magnesium

**What magnesium does**

Magnesium plays a significant role in neuromuscular balance and the regulation of neurotransmitters involved in relaxation and sleep. It helps the nervous system shift out of a heightened sympathetic state and supports deeper, more restorative sleep cycles.

**Why long-term stress affects magnesium.**

Stress increases urinary magnesium loss. The more prolonged the stress, the greater the depletion tends to be. Low magnesium levels can make it harder to relax into sleep or stay asleep.

**Signs you may be low.**

- Muscle tension or tightness
- Eye twitches or facial muscle flickers
- Difficulty winding down in the evening
- Restless sleep
- Headaches related to tension.

**When supplementation is useful**

For people experiencing sleep disruption linked to prolonged stress, magnesium can help restore neuromuscular calm and support more restful sleep.

## 2. Calcium

**What calcium does**

Calcium plays a role in muscle contraction/relaxation cycles and in the communication between nerves. It is involved in supporting sleep onset and maintaining stable sleep patterns.

**Why long-term stress affects calcium.**

Chronic stress can alter calcium metabolism indirectly through changes in cortisol and magnesium balance. When calcium and magnesium are out of sync, sleep can feel fragmented.

**Signs you may be low.**

- Difficulty settling the muscles at night
- Mild cramping (non-pathological)
- Feeling "restless" in the limbs
- Trouble staying asleep.

### When supplementation is useful

Calcium is best supported through a combined recalibration of magnesium and vitamin D. Supplementation can be helpful when intake is low, or if the balance between minerals has been disrupted by ongoing stress.

## 3. Vitamin D

### What vitamin D does

Vitamin D is involved in the regulation of circadian rhythms and sleep quality. Research shows a strong association between low vitamin D levels and sleep disturbances, including fragmented sleep, shorter duration, and poorer subjective sleep quality.

### Why long-term stress affects vitamin D.

Chronic stress may indirectly contribute to lower vitamin D levels by affecting behaviours such as time outdoors, appetite, and immune function. Vitamin D also interacts with pathways involved in inflammation, which can influence sleep patterns.

### Signs you may be low.

- Non-restorative sleep
- Waking frequently through the night
- Daytime tiredness
- General low mood that affects sleep quality.

### When supplementation is useful

Vitamin D supplementation can help restore sleep quality where a deficiency is present. Assessment through blood testing is recommended before commencing supplementation.

## 4. Vitamin B6

### What vitamin B6 does

Vitamin B6 plays a role in the production of serotonin and melatonin, neurotransmitters that are important for sleep regulation. Adequate levels help maintain normal sleep–wake cycles and support relaxation.

### Why long-term stress affects B6.

Stress increases metabolic demand for B6 because it is used in neurotransmitter synthesis. Over time, this can reduce availability for sleep-related pathways.

### Signs you may be low.

- Vivid dreams or night waking
- Difficulty relaxing before bed
- Low mood or irritability affecting sleep
- Feeling "wired but tired".

### When supplementation is useful

Supplementation may help individuals whose sleep difficulties relate to prolonged stress, low mood, or reduced serotonin synthesis. B6 is often used as part of a combined approach with magnesium.

## 5. Zinc

### What zinc does

Zinc is involved in supporting sleep architecture. It interacts with GABA and NMDA receptors, which help maintain a calmer nervous system and more consolidated sleep.

**Why long-term stress affects zinc.**

Stress can deplete zinc through altered immune activity and increased metabolic demand. Low zinc may contribute to difficulty with sleep onset, or poor sleep depth.

**Signs you may be low.**

- Light, easily disrupted sleep
- Frequent night waking
- Slower wound healing (suggestive of low zinc more broadly)
- Reduced appetite or changes in taste perception.

**When supplementation is useful**

A zinc supplement may support sleep quality where low levels are suspected or confirmed. It is often combined with magnesium or vitamin B6 as part of a broader sleep-support plan.

## 6. Iron

**What iron does**

Iron is crucial for oxygen transport, energy production, and neurological function. Its strongest link to sleep is through **restless legs syndrome (RLS)** and periodic limb movements, which can significantly disrupt sleep.

**Why long-term stress affects iron.**

Stress may influence iron through dietary patterns, inflammation, or changes in digestive function. Low iron is not directly caused by stress alone, but many people under prolonged strain have reduced intake or absorption.

**Signs you may be low.**

- Fatigue that isn't resolved by sleep
- Feeling cold or low in energy.

**When supplementation is useful**

Iron supplementation is only appropriate following a confirmed deficiency via blood testing. When deficiency-driven limb movement is present, correcting iron often significantly improves sleep quality.

## 15.4 - Digestive Support Nutrients

Long-term stress affects more than mood and sleep. It has well-documented effects on digestion. The gut is highly responsive to the stress response because it is directly regulated by the autonomic nervous system. When the body lives in fight-or-flight for extended periods - whether from burnout, chronic interpersonal stress, or prolonged exposure to destabilising behaviour - digestion can become irregular or uncomfortable.

Research shows that stress can alter gut motility, sensitivity, secretions, and even aspects of the gut barrier (Leigh et al., 2023; Konturek et al., 2011; Harvard Health Publishing, 2019). These shifts are biological, not psychological, and can happen even when someone feels they are "coping."

This chapter outlines **nutrients that support digestive function** because of their known roles in gut physiology. They do **not** reverse trauma, nor are they a treatment in isolation, but they can help the digestive system recover when stress has been high for a long time.

## 1. B Vitamins - Supporting Energy, Nerve Signalling and Cell Repair

### What they do

The B-group vitamins work across energy production, nerve function, and cellular repair. Several of them (particularly B6, folate, B12) support the normal turnover of intestinal cells and help maintain balanced immune activity in the gut (Hossain et al., 2022; Yang et al., 2025).

### How stress affects them

Stress can affect dietary intake, absorption, metabolism and gut microbiota composition, all of which can influence B-vitamin status (Pham et al., 2021).

### Possible deficiency-related symptoms

(Not diagnostic, simply patterns seen in deficiency research.)

- Low energy
- Poor concentration
- Mouth ulcers or sore tongue
- Heightened stress sensitivity
- In some cases, IBS-like symptoms have been associated with low B6 intake (Yang et al., 2025).

### Food sources

Whole grains, legumes, nuts, leafy vegetables, eggs, dairy, meat.

### Why they matter.

People recovering from chronic stress or destabilising environments often present with **fatigue, poor appetite and disrupted digestion**, and the B vitamins support the metabolic pathways involved in healing and restoration.

## 2. Vitamin D - Immune Modulation and Gut Barrier Support

### What it does

Vitamin D interacts with immune cells in the gut and supports normal barrier integrity through activation of the vitamin D receptor (VDR) in intestinal tissue (Akimbekov et al., 2020).

Supplementation in deficient adults has been shown to positively influence gut microbial composition and diversity (Singh et al., 2020; Malaguarnera et al., 2020).

### How stress affects vitamin D

People under chronic stress may experience:

- Reduced sunlight exposure
- Decreased outdoor time
- Disrupted diet

- all of which can contribute to low vitamin D.

### Possible deficiency signs

- Fatigue
- Low mood
- Higher susceptibility to infections
- Muscle aches.

### Food sources

Oily fish, eggs, fortified foods; safe sunlight.

**Why it matters.**

Immune changes and gut disruption often occur during prolonged relational stress. Vitamin D supports the **immune-gut axis,** which is relevant when the body is trying to stabilise.

## 3. Zinc - Repairing Gut Tissue and Supporting Immune Function

**What it does**

Zinc contributes to:

- Intestinal barrier integrity
- Mucosal repair
- Balanced immune responses in the digestive tract.

These effects are documented in human and preclinical research (Skrovanek et al., 2014; Wan et al., 2022; Wang et al., 2024).

**How stress affects zinc status**

Chronic stress can alter appetite and digestion. Gut inflammation or dysbiosis can also reduce zinc absorption or increase utilisation.

**Possible deficiency signs**

- Reduced appetite
- Poor wound healing
- Changes in taste and smell
- More frequent infections.

**Food sources**

Pumpkin seeds, meat, poultry, seafood, legumes.

**Why it matters.**

For people experiencing digestive disruption during or after abusive or high-stress environments, zinc may support the structural repair of the gut lining and immune balance.

## 4. Vitamin E - Antioxidant Support for Gut Tissue

**What vitamin E does**

Vitamin E is a fat-soluble antioxidant. In preclinical studies it:

- Reduces oxidative stress in intestinal tissue
- May support barrier function under conditions of physiological stress.

These effects are seen in models of intestinal injury or inflammation (Wang et al., 2020; Wu et al., 2024).

When combined with selenium, vitamin E has demonstrated protective effects on gut tissue in experimental settings (Liu et al., 2016).

**Why it matters.**

Oxidative stress and inflammatory signalling are heightened during long-term psychological stress. Supporting antioxidant capacity may help the gut as part of broader recovery.

**Food sources**

Nuts, seeds, vegetable oils, whole grains.

## 5. Probiotics

The gut microbiota plays a major role in:

- Immune tolerance
- Digestion
- Inflammation
- Communication with the nervous system.

Stress can alter gut microbiota composition (Konturek et al., 2011; Warren et al., 2024).

Certain probiotic strains have shown benefits for:

- IBS symptom improvement
- Gut inflammation
- Immune regulation
- Improving oral tolerance, particularly in children (Ma et al., 2019; Di Costanzo et al., 2024; Tordesillas et al., 2018).

There is **no evidence** that probiotics specifically reverse the digestive effects of narcissistic abuse. They are a digestive support option, not trauma treatment.

### Why they matter.

People with long-term relational stress often present with disrupted digestion. Probiotics may support gut comfort, motility and immune balance, depending on the strain.

This should always be practitioner-guided.

### A Note on Stress and Digestive Symptoms

The digestive consequences of stress can include:

- Constipation

- Diarrhoea
- Alternating bowel patterns
- Bloating
- Nausea
- Abdominal discomfort
- Increased gut sensitivity.

These changes are mediated through the gut–brain axis. They are **physiological**, not "in your head." And they commonly begin to settle once the stress load reduces, with additional improvement when nutritional status is restored. Always consult your qualified health care professional to determine if there's an underlying physiological condition that also needs attention.

### 15.5 - Herbal Medicines for Nervous System Stability

A tool that I find to be of benefit with bringing the body back into balance is herbal medicine. A qualified herbalist is able to make you a specific, tailored blend to suit you and provide additional complementary medicine support.

In this section I've also included technical data for health care professionals. It's by no means exhaustive; it gives further information as a reference.

**Always consult your qualified health care professional to determine if there's an underlying physiological condition that also needs attention whenever you are experiencing symptoms and never self-prescribe.**

## SECTION 1A - Nervines (Herbs That Calm an Overactive Nervous System)

When people have been chronically stressed, overwhelmed, or living in environments where they've spent years being hypervigilant, the nervous system can feel like it's running on several unstable channels at once.

Nervine herbs support the nervous system's return to steadier functioning.
They don't "fix" anything and they don't override physiology, but they do help nudge the system towards balance, so the body can do what it is trying very hard to do on its own.

These herbs differ in action: some calm, some soothe digestive tension, some support sleep onset, and some help soften the physical sensation of bracing.

Below are the **primary evidence-based nervines**, grouped with dual-format explanations.

### 1. *Matricaria chamomilla* / *Matricaria recutita* (Chamomile)

**What it does**

Chamomile is one of the most well-researched calming herbs. It acts on the nervous system through mild GABA-modulating effects, which help reduce physical tension and support a calmer emotional baseline. It also helps settle digestive upsets triggered by stress (the gut–brain axis in action).

Some benefits may be:

- Reduced muscle tension
- Less digestive cramping
- Gentler emotional reactivity
- Improved ability to wind down.

Chamomile is especially supportive for people whose stress shows up as both **gut symptoms and nervous irritability at the same time**.

### Why it helps under stress.

Chronic stress reduces GABA activity and increases sympathetic drive.
Chamomile contains apigenin, which interacts with GABA receptors in a mild, non-sedative way, helping the system shift out of continual activation.

### Symptoms that may shift

- Stress-related indigestion
- Restlessness
- Difficulty calming before sleep.

### Cross-system overlap

- Digestive support through mild bitter actions
- Anti-inflammatory effects in the gut mucosa
- Mild antispasmodic activity.

### Clinician note.

- Avoid if allergic to Asteraceae (Daisy) family
- Very well tolerated in most people
- Apigenin acts on benzodiazepine receptors (non-addictive)
- ESCOP monograph supports anxiolytic, spasmolytic effects
- No significant CYP450 interactions reported.

## References

Amsterdam, J. D., Li, Y., Soeller, I., Rockwell, K., Mao, J. J., & Shults, J. (2009). A randomized, double-blind, placebo-controlled trial of oral chamomile extract in generalized anxiety disorder. *Journal of Clinical Psychopharmacology*, 29(4), 378–382.

Srivastava, J. K., Shankar, E., & Gupta, S. (2010). Chamomile: A herbal medicine of the past with bright future (Review). *Molecular Medicine Reports*, 3(6), 895–901.

ESCOP Monographs: *Matricariae flos*.

## 2. *Lavandula angustifolia* (Lavender — Herb and Essential Oil)

**What it does**

Lavender has measurable calming effects on the nervous system - not anecdotal but repeatedly demonstrated in clinical trials. The essential oil (inhaled or oral standardised extract) has the strongest anxiolytic (helps the symptoms associated with mild anxiety) data.

**Why it helps under stress.**

Lavender interacts with serotonin and GABA pathways, supporting the shift out of sympathetic overdrive.

**Symptoms that may shift**

- Nervous agitation
- Stress-related headaches
- Sleep-onset difficulties
- Irritability.

## Cross-system overlap

- Mild analgesic activity
- Supports parasympathetic tone.

## Clinician note.

- Generally, well tolerated
- Essential oil should not be ingested unless in a clinically tested formulation
- Topical reactions are rare, but possible
- Oral *Silexan* (standardized lavender extract) demonstrated non-sedative anxiolytic activity with effect sizes comparable to low-dose benzodiazepines (Kasper, 2010)
- No withdrawal or dependence risk documented.

## References

Kasper, S., et al. (2010). Lavender oil preparation Silexan is effective in GAD. *International Journal of Psychiatry in Clinical Practice*, 14(3), 243–249.

Woelk, H., & Schläfke, S. (2010). A multi-center study of a lavender oil preparation vs. lorazepam. *Phytomedicine*, 17(2), 94–99.

ESCOP Monographs: *Lavandulae aetheroleum*.

### 3. *Melissa officinalis* (Lemon Balm)

#### What it does

Lemon balm supports people who might be mentally busy, or easily overstimulated.
It has gentle calming activity and can help improve focus when anxiety or overthinking is getting in the way.

**Why it helps under stress.**

Lemon balm influences GABA activity and reduces stress-induced agitation.
It has also shown improvements in cognitive performance, when the nervous system is overloaded.

**Symptoms that may shift**

- Nervous tension
- Digestive tension linked with stress.

- **Cross-system overlap**

- Mild carminative and antispasmodic activity
- Supports digestive symptoms linked with stress.

**Clinician note.**

- 300 mg extracts reduced stress-induced negative mood and improved calmness in controlled trials (Kennedy, 2004)
- Well-tolerated generally
- Avoid large doses in hypothyroidism, without practitioner guidance.

**References**

Kennedy, D. O., et al. (2004). Effects of *Melissa officinalis* on mood and cognitive performance. *Pharmacology Biochemistry and Behavior*, 79(2), 373–384.

ESCOP Monographs: *Melissae folium.*

## 4. *Passiflora incarnata* (Passionflower)

### What it does

Passionflower is useful for mild sleep issues. It has a calming effect, without sedation and stress-related restlessness.

### Why it helps under stress.

It modulates GABAergic activity, reducing hyperexcitability. Often suited to individuals who "can't switch off."

### Symptoms that may shift

- Pre-sleep restlessness
- Nervous tension
- Physical agitation.

### Cross-system overlap

- Mild antispasmodic effects.

### Clinician note.

- Generally, well tolerated
- Not recommended in pregnancy
- Comparable anxiolytic efficacy to oxazepam in small trials without sedative or dependency risk (Akhondzadeh, 2001).

### References

Akhondzadeh, S., et al. (2001). Passionflower in GAD: A pilot study. *Journal of Clinical Pharmacy and Therapeutics*, 26(5), 363–367.

ESCOP Monographs: *Passiflorae herba*.

## 5. *Scutellaria lateriflora* (Skullcap)

### What it does

Skullcap supports nervous system overstimulation. People often describe the effect as "taking the edge off" without drowsiness.

### Why it helps under stress.

Its flavonoids interact with GABA receptors, helping reduce muscular and mental tension.

### Cross-system overlap

- Mild analgesic actions.

### Clinician note.

- Ensure products are authentic (historical adulteration issues)
- Generally well-tolerated
- No major interactions reported
- Use caution in hepatic disease (historical concern with adulterants only).

### References

Wills, R. B., Bone, K., & Morgan, M. (2000). Herbal medicines: *Scutellaria lateriflora* review. *Journal of Herbal Pharmacotherapy*.

ESCOP Monographs.

## 6. *Leonurus cardiaca* (Motherwort)

### What it does

Motherwort calms the nervous system **and** the cardiovascular system and is helpful when stress presents as palpitations or a racing heart.

### Why it helps under stress.

It supports parasympathetic activity and has mild hypotensive and anxiolytic effects.

### Symptoms that may shift

- Stress-related palpitations
- Irritability
- PMS-related nervous tension.

### Cross-system overlap

- Cardiovascular support
- Menstrual tension support.

### Clinician note.

- Avoid in pregnancy due to uterine-stimulating effects
- Contains leonurine with documented cardiotonic activity
- Mild MAO-inhibiting effect (theoretical, somonitor with antidepressants).

### References

Blumenthal, M. (Ed.). (2003). *The ABC Clinical Guide to Herbs.*

ESCOP Monographs: *Leonuri cardiacae herba.*

## SECTION 1B - Adaptogens

Adaptogens are herbs that help the body adjust to stress more effectively.
They don't force stimulation or sedation. Instead, they support the physiological systems involved in stress responses, particularly the HPA axis, immune modulation, inflammatory signalling, and energy regulation.

Crucially: **Adaptogens don't "fix" trauma, abuse, or emotional wounds. They support the physical body while you stabilise.** That's their role - to reduce the physiological load, so the nervous system isn't fighting on every front at once.

Below are the adaptogens with **robust evidence** and **strong relevance** to post-stress recovery.

### 1. *Withania somnifera* (Ashwagandha)

*(Primary action: adaptogen, anxiolytic, sleep support)*

### What it does

Ashwagandha is one of the most well-researched adaptogens for reducing stress-related physiological load. People often describe feeling "more level," "less reactive," or "not running on adrenaline all day."

Clinically demonstrated actions include:

- Supporting cortisol regulation
- Reducing perceived stress
- Improving sleep onset and sleep quality
- Supporting energy without overstimulation.

### Why it helps under chronic stress.

Chronic hypervigilance and ongoing relational stress elevate cortisol and activate several inflammatory pathways. Ashwagandha supports HPA axis recalibration, helping the system re-establish a more stable hormonal baseline.

### Symptoms that may shift

- Constant tension
- Poor sleep
- Morning fatigue
- Stress-induced inflammation
- Irritability.

### Cross-system overlap

- Mild thyroid support (T4 → T3 conversion)
- Anti-inflammatory activity
- Immune modulation.

### Clinician note.

Do **not** use in:

- Hyperthyroidism (unless under supervision)
- Pregnancy
- Nightshade family allergies.
- Multiple RCTs show significant reductions in cortisol (Chandrasekhar et al., 2012)
- Sedative-withdrawal support has been documented in some observational data
- Immune-modulating activity via withanolides.

### References

Chandrasekhar, K., Kapoor, J., & Anishetty, S. (2012). A prospective, randomized double-blind, placebo-controlled study of safety and efficacy of a high-concentration ashwagandha root extract. *Indian Journal of Psychological Medicine*, 34(3), 255–262.

Lopresti, A. (2022). Ashwagandha in stress and anxiety. *Journal of Clinical Medicine*, 11(2).

Braun, L., & Cohen, M. (2015). *Herbs & Natural Supplements* (4th ed.).

## 2. *Schisandra chinensis* (Schisandra)

*(Primary action: adaptogen, hepatoprotective, neuroprotective)*

### What it does

Schisandra helps stabilise energy, sharpen mental clarity, and build resilience to ongoing stress. It tends to be "balancing" rather than sedating and is used for stress recovery. and overstimulation alternate.

### Why it helps under chronic stress.

Chronic dysregulation affects liver detoxification, mitochondrial function, and inflammatory signalling. Schisandra supports these systems, which can lift the background "drag" caused by prolonged stress.

### Symptoms that may shift

- Brain fog
- Low daytime stamina
- Fatigue with poor endurance.

### Cross-system overlap

- Liver support (evidence-based)
- Antioxidant effects

- Mild anxiolytic (helps with symptoms of mild anxiety) activity.

**Clinician note.**

Avoid in:

- Acute hepatitis
- Pregnancy (limited data)
- Lignans (schisandrin A/B/C) demonstrated hepatoprotective and adaptogenic effects in several trials.
- Animal and limited human data show improvements in stress tolerance
- CYP450 interactions possible (CYP3A4, CYP2E1).

**References**

Panossian, A., & Wikman, G. (2008). Pharmacology of Schisandra. *Phytomedicine*, 15(9), 833–848.

Henderson, L., Yue, Q., & Bergner, P. (2005). *The Healing Power of Schisandra.*

ESCOP Monographs: *Schisandrae chinensis fructus.*

### 3. *Ocimum tenuiflorum / O. sanctum* (Holy Basil / Tulsi)

*(Primary action: adaptogen, anxiolytic, anti-inflammatory)*

**What it does**

Holy basil supports mood, stress tolerance, and immune support. Holy basil helps regulate cortisol, supports antioxidant activity, and has mild mood-stabilising effects in clinical studies.

## Cross-system overlap

- Anti-inflammatory
- Antioxidant
- Digestive calming effects.

## Clinician note.

Avoid in:

- Pregnancy
- People taking anticoagulants (theoretical interaction)
- Human studies show reductions in stress scores, cortisol, and improved cognitive performance (Jamshidi & Cohen, 2017)
- May support metabolic markers under stress.

## References

Jamshidi, N., & Cohen, M. (2017). The clinical efficacy of Tulsi. *Journal of Ayurveda and Integrative Medicine*, 8(1), 66–75.

Braun, L., & Cohen, M. (2015). *Herbs & Natural Supplements* (4th ed.).

## 4. *Bacopa monnieri* (Bacopa)

*(Primary action: adaptogen-like nootropic, cognitive support)*

## What it does

Bacopa supports memory, information processing, and focus. Long-term stress impacts the hippocampus and neurotransmitter balance.
Bacopa has strong evidence for supporting memory, speed of learning, and cognitive resilience under pressure.

### Symptoms that may shift

- Brain fog
- Difficulty concentrating
- Poor recall
- Mental fatigue.

### Cross-system overlap

- Mild anxiolytic effects
- Antioxidant activity.

### Clinician note.

- May cause mild digestive discomfort in some people
- Avoid in pregnancy
- Bacosides improve synaptic communication and support hippocampal function
- Significant evidence base for cognitive enhancement (Stough et al., 2001; Pase et al., 2012).

### References

Pase, M. P., Kean, J., Sarris, J., et al. (2012). The cognitive-enhancing effects of Bacopa. *Journal of Alternative and Complementary Medicine*, 18(7), 647–653.

Stough, C., Lloyd, J., Clarke, J., et al. (2001). The chronic effects of Bacopa on cognition. *Psychopharmacology*, 156(4), 481–484.

ESCOP Monographs: *Bacopa monnieri herba*.

### 5. *Crocus sativus* (Saffron)

*(Primary action: mood support, mild adaptogenic activity)*

**What it does**

Saffron has robust evidence for improving mood, reducing low motivation, and supporting emotional recovery after long-term stress.
It works gently but steadily - not stimulating, not sedating.

**Why it helps under chronic stress.**

Saffron influences serotonin modulation, reduces neuroinflammation, and supports oxidative balance, all of can be dysregulated under prolonged stress.

**Cross-system overlap**

- Antioxidant
- Supports cognitive function.

**Clinician note.**

- Avoid during pregnancy
- Therapeutic extracts are generally well tolerated
- Multiple RCTs show saffron comparable to SSRIs for mild-to-moderate depression
- Crocin and safranal are primary active constituents.

**References**

Hausenblas, H. A., et al. (2015). Saffron in mood improvement: meta-analysis. *Human Psychopharmacology*, 30(2), 102–111.

Toth, B., et al. (2019). Saffron and depression. *Frontiers in Nutrition*, 6, 3.

## SECTION 1C – Multifunctional Nervous System Herbs

This group of herbs primarily support the nervous system, but also influence other areas such as sleep, mild pain modulation, emotional steadiness, digestive tension, or muscle relaxation.

These are not sedatives in the pharmaceutical sense. They work by easing hyperarousal, supporting parasympathetic activity, or reducing the internal "load" that shows up after chronic relational stress.

### 1. *Ziziphus jujuba var. spinosa* (Zizyphus)

*(Primary actions: anxiolytic, hypnotic, nervous system stabiliser)*

**What it does**

Zizyphus is widely used in Chinese medicine for calming an overactive mind, reducing nighttime agitation, and supporting deeper, more restorative sleep.

**Symptoms that may shift**

- Disturbed and restless sleep

**Cross-system overlap**

- Mild digestive calming
- Antioxidant effects.

**Clinician note.**

Generally well tolerated.
Avoid in:

- Pregnancy (lack of robust data)

- Jujubosides modulate GABA_A receptors (Zhang et al., 2003)
- RCTs show improvements in sleep quality and latency
- May potentiate CNS depressants (theoretical).

## References

Chen, C., et al. (2014). Suan Zao Ren and insomnia: clinical trial review. *Phytomedicine*, 21(7), 914–922.

Zhang, R., et al. (2003). Jujubosides and GABA modulation. *Journal of Ethnopharmacology*, 89(2–3), 99–102.

ESCOP Monographs: *Zizyphi spinosae semen*.

## 2. *Valeriana officinalis* (Valerian)

*(Primary actions: anxiolytic, mild sedative, sleep support)*

### What it does

Valerian is best known for helping people fall asleep more easily, but it also reduces nervous tension during the day.

### Why it helps under chronic stress

Valerian supports GABA activity - the neurotransmitter associated with calming and regulating the nervous system. It helps counter the "on edge" physiology that builds under persistent relational stress.

### Symptoms that may shift

- Difficulty falling asleep
- Restlessness
- Stress-driven muscle tension

- Irritability.

**Cross-system overlap**

- Mild analgesic effects (evidence-supported)
- Muscle relaxation
- Gentle antispasmodic activity.

**Clinician note.**

Avoid:

- Combining with alcohol
- Operating machinery, until you understand your response
- Valerenic acids modulate GABA_A receptors
- Some trials show equivalency to benzodiazepines for mild anxiety, though results vary
- CYP450 interactions possible, but generally low risk.

**References**

Sultana, J., et al. (2018). Valerian and sleep: systematic review. *Sleep Medicine Reviews*, 38, 175–185.

Fernandez-San-Martin, M. I., et al. (2010). Valerian for insomnia: meta-analysis. *American Journal of Medicine*, 123(4), 276.e9–276.e15.

Braun, L., & Cohen, M. (2015). *Herbs & Natural Supplements*.

### 3. *Eschscholzia californica* (California poppy)

*(Primary actions: anxiolytic, sedative, mild analgesic)*

## What it does

California poppy helps support sleep. California poppy acts through GABA pathways and mild opioid receptor modulation (non-addictive), supporting calming and comfort.

## Cross-system overlap

- Gentle analgesic action
- Mild antispasmodic activity.

## Clinician note.

Avoid in:

- Pregnancy
- Concurrent sedative medications unless supervised
- Contains protopine and allocryptopine with CNS-modulating activity
- RCTs show anxiolytic and sedative synergy when combined with other nervines.

## References

Rolland, A., et al. (1991). Sedative and anxiolytic effects of California poppy. *Planta Medica*, 57(3), 212–216.

ESCOP Monographs: *Eschscholzia californica herba*.

## SECTION 1D - Sleep Focused Herbs

Sleep tends to be one of the last areas to settle after long-term relational stress.
These herbs have evidence for:

- Reducing night-time arousal
- Supporting sleep onset
- Improving sleep quality
- Reducing the agitation, looped thoughts, or physiological hypervigilance that interfere with sleep.

This section covers herbs **not already detailed** in earlier nervous-system chapters.

### 1. *Passiflora incarnata* (Passionflower)

*(Primary actions: anxiolytic, sedative, supports sleep onset)*

### What it does

Passionflower helps quieten mental overactivity, particularly at night.
It's useful when the mind loops or overthinks, or when you feel tired, but can't "drop down" into sleep.

Some benefits may be:

- Easier transition into sleep

### Why it helps under chronic stress.

Prolonged stress increases physiological arousal and disrupts GABA signalling.
Passionflower supports GABA activity, helping the system shift toward rest-and-repair.

## Symptoms that may shift

- Difficulty falling asleep
- Light, easily broken sleep.

## Cross-system overlap

- Mild digestive calming
- Gentle antispasmodic effects.

Avoid or seek supervision if:

- Taking sedatives
- Pregnant (insufficient safety data)
- Flavonoids such as chrysin show GABAergic modulation
- RCTs show improvement in sleep quality in mild insomnia and anxiety populations
- Generally safe with SSRIs/SNRIs, though caution is advised due to sedative synergy.

## References

Ngan, A., & Conduit, R. (2011). Passionflower and sleep quality: RCT. *Phytotherapy Research*, 25(8), 1153–1159.

Akhondzadeh, S., et al. (2001). Passionflower vs. oxazepam for anxiety. *Journal of Clinical Pharmacy and Therapeutics*, 26(5), 363–367.

ESCOP Monographs: *Passiflorae herba*.

## 3. *Melissa officinalis* (Lemon balm)

*(Primary actions: anxiolytic, sleep-supportive, digestive-nervous interface)*

## What it does

Lemon balm is for people whose sleep is affected by emotional tension, digestive discomfort, or low-grade symptoms associated with mild anxiety.
It's gentle and stabilising, with good evidence for reducing nervous irritability.

Some benefits may be:

- Calmer evenings
- Easier sleep onset
- Reduced "tummy tension" linked to stress.

## Why it helps under chronic stress.

Lemon balm affects both the nervous system and the gut–brain axis.
Research shows GABA-transaminase inhibition, which supports calm and improves sleep quality.

## Cross-system overlap

- Digestive calming (carminative action)
- Mild cognitive benefits (short-term stress performance trials).

## Clinician note.

Generally well tolerated.

Use with care in:

- Hypothyroidism (theoretical - largely outdated but still referenced)
- Rosmarinic acid inhibits GABA-T

- RCTs show improvements in sleep quality, anxiety, and stress-related symptoms
- No significant interactions documented at therapeutic doses.

**References**

Cases, J., et al. (2011). Melissa officinalis for stress and anxiety: RCT. *Mediterranean Journal of Nutrition and Metabolism*, 4(3), 211–218.

Kennedy, D. O., et al. (2004). Lemon balm and cognitive performance. *Psychosomatic Medicine*, 66(4), 607–613.

ESCOP Monographs: *Melissae folium.*

**Immune–Stress Adaptation Herbs**

This section is in a slightly different format; a practitioner will need to determine which, if any, immune-stress adaptation herbs might suit you best.

Chronic relational stress can affect immune function, not because someone is "weak," but because long-term activation of the stress response reshapes inflammatory pathways, cytokine signalling, and immune cell activity (Segerstrom & Miller, 2004; Dhabhar, 2014; Cohen et al., 2012).

Herbs in this section do **not** "boost" immunity. They **modulate** it - nudging it back toward balance.

**1 *Eleutherococcus senticosus* (Siberian ginseng /Eleuthero)**

Eleuthero is traditionally used as an adaptogen - a herb that helps the body cope with stress. Research also shows that it can influence parts of the immune system, particularly NK cells and T-cell activity, especially under stress conditions.

After long-term emotional or relational strain, eleuthero may support:

- Day-to-day resilience
- Immune steadiness during ongoing stress
- Energy regulation under pressure.

It is stimulating for some people, so clinician guidance is recommended.

**Clinician note.**

- Evidence of increased NK cell activity and modulation of T-cell responses in healthy adults under stress.
- Mechanisms: mild HPA axis modulation, catecholamine stabilisation, immunomodulation.
- Caution in hypertension, arrhythmias, insomnia; use carefully in autoimmune conditions.

**References — Eleuthero**

Panossian, A., & Wikman, G. (2010). *Pharmaceuticals*, *3*(1), 188–224.

Cicero, A. F. G., et al. (2004). *Journal of Ethnopharmacology*.

Davydov, M., & Krikorian, A. (2000). *J Ethnopharmacol.* (Review of adaptogenic activity).

## 2 *Echinacea* spp. (Echinacea)

Echinacea is widely recognised for respiratory immunity. Research shows that certain standardised extracts can modestly reduce the frequency and duration of respiratory infections, particularly relevant because chronic stress increases susceptibility.

It is not suitable for everyone, especially those with autoimmune conditions or significant allergies.

**Clinician note.**

- Meta-analyses show modest reduction in URTI incidence and duration (extract-specific).
- Mechanisms include macrophage activation, phagocytosis, cytokine modulation (TNF-α, IL-6), and endocannabinoid system interaction.
- Caution with autoimmune conditions and Asteraceae sensitivity.

**References — Echinacea**

Lee, M. S., et al. (2024). *Phytotherapy Research.*

Sumer, S., et al. (2023). *Frontiers in Medicine, 10.*

Melchart, D., et al. (1994). *Planta Medica.*

Woelkart, K., & Bauer, R. (2007). *International Immunopharmacology.*

## 3 *Ocimum tenuiflorum* / *O. sanctum* (Holy basil / Tulsi)

Holy basil has growing clinical research for:

- Reducing perceived stress
- Improving sleep quality
- Supporting immune and metabolic balance.

It also targets both nervous system tension and inflammatory pathways, which is useful after long-term stress.

**Clinician note.**

- RCTs show reduced stress, improved sleep, and improved attention with tulsi extracts.
- Mechanisms include NF-κB modulation, COX-2 inhibition, antioxidant activity, and influence on cortisol.
- Caution with anticoagulants, hypoglycaemics, and CYP-modulating medications.

**References — Holy basil**

Pradhan, D., et al. (2022). *Journal of Ethnopharmacology, 296.*

Cohen, M. M. (2014). *Journal of Ayurveda and Integrative Medicine.*

Mondal, S., et al. (2009). *Indian Journal of Physiology and Pharmacology.*

### 4 *Schisandra chinensis* (Schisandra)

Schisandra is traditionally used for fatigue, stress, and liver support. Modern research shows it:

- Supports antioxidant systems
- Modulates stress hormones
- Can influence immune responses indirectly, through liver and HPA effects.

### 5 *Albizia lebbeck* (Albizia)

Albizia has been used traditionally for allergies, skin conditions, and respiratory irritation. Research suggests it may:

- Stabilise mast cells
- Reduce inflammatory cytokines
- Decrease histamine release.

This is relevant where long-term stress has worsened inflammatory or allergic tendencies.

**Clinicians Note**

- Evidence of mast-cell stabilisation, reduced histamine release, and suppression of H1 receptor and histidine decarboxylase gene expression.
- Some clinical benefit demonstrated for allergic rhinitis and asthma (small trials).
- Use caution in autoimmune disease; insufficient pregnancy safety data.

**References — Albizia**

Nurul, I. M., et al. (2011). *International Immunopharmacology, 11*(11).

Sharma, V., et al. (2019). *Journal of Herbal Medicine.*

Kamboj, A., et al. (2017). *Journal of Ayurveda and Integrative Medicine.*

**Clinicians Note**

- Known for hepatic glutathione enhancement and antioxidant enzyme upregulation.
- Modulates stress-induced cortisol changes and inflammatory signalling.
- Use caution with CYP450 interactions; consider preparation-specific variability.

**References — Schisandra**

Panossian, A., & Wikman, G. (2010). *Pharmaceuticals, 3*(1).

Szopa, A., et al. (2017). *Phytochemistry Reviews.*

Hu, D. (2021). *Frontiers in Pharmacology.*

## 6 *Uncaria tomentosa* (Cat's claw)

Cat's claw is known for its **anti-inflammatory and immune-modulating** effects. It does not "boost" the immune system, rather it helps regulate overactive or dysregulated pathways.

This herb may be helpful when chronic stress has contributed to inflammatory symptoms.

## Clinician note.

- Demonstrated inhibition of NF-$\varkappa$B activation and reductions in TNF-$\alpha$, IL-1$\beta$, and IL-6.
- Some clinical evidence for osteoarthritis and inflammatory conditions.
- Strictly contraindicated in pregnancy; caution in autoimmune disease.

## References — Cat's claw

Sandoval, M., et al. (2000). *Journal of Ethnopharmacology*.

Piscoya, J., et al. (2001). *Inflammation Research*.

Keplinger, K., et al. (1999). *Journal of Natural Products*.

## 7 *Hericium erinaceus* (Lion's mane mushroom)

Lion's mane is widely used for cognitive and nervous system support, but it also has evidence for:

- Immune regulation
- Gut-associated immune activity
- Antioxidant support.

Some human studies show improvements in **sleep and mild anxiety**.

## Note for clinicians

- Polysaccharides activate macrophages, NK cells, and modulate gut immune tissue (MAPK, AKT signalling).
- Small human trials suggest benefits for mild cognitive impairment, anxiety, and sleep.
- Use caution with mushroom allergies and autoimmune conditions.

## References — Lion's mane

Liu, J., et al. (2022). *Food Chemistry: X, 13*, 100214.

Han, Y., et al. (2023). *Bioscience, Biotechnology, and Biochemistry, 87*(3).

Mori, K., et al. (2011). *Biomedical Research*.

## SECTION 2 - Digestive Herbs

*Matricaria chamomilla / Matricaria recutita* (German Chamomile)

*(Primary actions: digestive carminative, anti-inflammatory, mild anxiolytic, spasmolytic)*

### What it does

German chamomile is traditionally used for digestive tension - the kind that shows up when stress lands in the gut. It calms the smooth muscle of the GI tract, reduces bloating after meals, and supports people who experience abdominal discomfort when they're anxious.

Some benefits may be:
- Reduced digestive cramping
- Gentler digestion after eating
- Less "nervous stomach" tension
- Calmer mood, alongside digestive relief.

### Why it helps under chronic stress.

Chamomile's digestive benefits relate to its spasmolytic activity (apigenin + other flavonoids), which relaxes GI smooth muscle. It also shows mild anxiolytic activity through GABA-A receptor interactions - helpful when stress drives gut symptoms.

### Symptoms that may shift

- Stress-related bloating
- Upper abdominal discomfort
- Digestive "tightness" linked to worry.

## Cross-system overlap

- Mild nervous-system calming
- Sleep support (in some individuals)
- Local anti-inflammatory effects in the gut mucosa.

## Clinician note.

Very well tolerated.

Considerations:
- Asteraceae family allergy risk (rare but documented)
- Mild anticoagulant potential due to coumarin content (theoretical; not typically clinically significant).

Mechanisms and findings:
- Apigenin shows smooth-muscle relaxation in GI models
- RCTs demonstrate chamomile reducing functional dyspepsia symptoms
- Anti-inflammatory effects observed via COX-2 and nitric oxide modulation.

## References

Amsterdam, J. D., et al. (2009). Chamomile for generalized anxiety disorder. *J Clin Psychopharmacol,* 29(4), 378–382.

ESCOP Monographs: *Chamomillae flos.*

McKay, D. L., & Blumberg, J. B. (2006). A review of the bioactivity of chamomile tea. *Phytother Res,* 20, 519–530.

Srivastava, J. K., et al. (2010). Chamomile: phytochemical constituents and therapeutic uses. *Mol Med Report,* 3(6), 895–901.

## *Zingiber officinale* (Ginger)

*(Primary actions: anti-inflammatory, pro-kinetic, anti-nausea, digestive stimulant)*

### What it does

Ginger supports digestion, where stress contributes to slowed motility, nausea, or bloating.
It helps stimulate digestive secretions and reduces upper-gut discomfort.

Some benefits may be:
• Reduced nausea
• Less bloating
• Easier digestion after meals
• A sense of warmth.

### Symptoms that may shift

• Nausea
• Sluggish digestion
• Early fullness
• Post-meal bloating.

### Cross-system overlap

• Anti-inflammatory activity
• Mild analgesic effects.

### Clinician note.

Generally well tolerated.

Use with care in:
• Gallstones (due to cholagogic activity)
• People on anticoagulants (theoretical, dose-dependent; human RCTs show minimal interaction).

Mechanisms and findings:
- 6-gingerol and shogaols modulate serotonin receptors involved in nausea pathways
- RCTs show improved gastric emptying in functional dyspepsia
- Significant anti-inflammatory activity via NF-κB downregulation.

## References

Borrelli, F., et al. (2005). Ginger and GI motility. *Phytother Res*, *19*(9), 695–699.

Lete, I., & Allué, J. (2016). Ginger for nausea/vomiting. *Nutrients*, *8*(11), 761.

ESCOP Monographs: *Zingiberis rhizoma*.

## *Mentha × piperita* (Peppermint)

*(Primary actions: antispasmodic, carminative, pro-motility, analgesic for GI discomfort)*

### What it does

Peppermint is one of the most well-studied herbs for digestive tension and IBS-type symptoms.
It relaxes the smooth muscle of the intestines, reduces spasms, and eases gas-related discomfort.

Some benefits may be:
- Less cramping
- Easier digestion
- Reduced gas and bloating.

## Why it helps under chronic stress.

Stress increases GI muscle tension and can slow or disrupt motility.
Peppermint's menthol relaxes smooth muscle via calcium channel blockade, helping the gut move more freely.

## Symptoms that may shift

- Abdominal cramping
- IBS-pattern pain
- Gas and bloating
- Post-meal discomfort.

## Cross-system overlap

- Mild analgesic effects

## Clinician note.

Generally well tolerated.

Considerations:
- May worsen reflux in some due to relaxation of the lower oesophageal sphincter
- Enteric-coated formulations used in RCTs for IBS
- Not for infants (risk of laryngospasm from menthol vapour).

Mechanisms and findings:
- Menthol blocks calcium channels → smooth muscle relaxation
- RCTs consistently show reductions in pain and global IBS symptoms
- Comparable efficacy to some antispasmodic medications.

## References

Cash, B. D., et al. (2016). Peppermint oil and IBS. *Digestive Diseases and Sciences, 61*(2), 560–571.*

Ford, A. C., et al. (2008). Effectiveness of peppermint oil in IBS — systematic review. *BMJ, 337*, a2313.

ESCOP Monographs: *Menthae piperitae aetheroleum.*

### *Foeniculum vulgare* (Fennel)

*(Primary actions: carminative, antispasmodic, anti-inflammatory, digestive relaxant)*

### What it does

Fennel is used for bloating, digestive tightness, and spasmodic discomfort.
It's gentle and helpful when stress leads to upper or lower GI wind and tension.

Some benefits may be:
- Reduced bloating
- Easier passage of gas
- Less gripping abdominal tension.

### Why it helps under chronic stress.

Stress increases motility dysregulation and aerophagia (air swallowing).
Fennel relaxes smooth muscle and improves gas dispersion.

### Symptoms that may shift

- Bloating
- Spasmodic lower abdominal pain
- Stress-associated wind
- Functional digestive discomfort.

## Cross-system overlap

- Mild galactagogue activity (traditional; not the focus here)
- Anti-inflammatory action via anethole.

## Clinician note.

Generally well tolerated.

*Considerations:*
*• Avoid in people with known celery/mugwort allergies (rare cross-reactivity)*
*• Theoretical oestrogenic concerns largely unsupported at dietary/therapeutic doses.*

Mechanisms and findings:
- Anethole exhibits smooth-muscle–relaxing effects
- RCTs show symptom reductions in functional dyspepsia and IBS
- Anti-inflammatory activity enhances mucosal comfort.

## References

Portincasa, P., et al. (2016). Fennel for functional digestive symptoms. *Eur Rev Med Pharmacol Sci, 20,* 558–563.

Badgujar, S. B., et al. (2014). Fennel phytochemistry and biomedicine. *BioMed Research International, 2014,* 842674.

ESCOP Monographs: *Foeniculi fructus.*

## *Cynara scolymus* (Globe artichoke)

*(Primary actions: choleretic, cholekinetic, digestive stimulant, anti-dyspeptic)*

## What it does

Artichoke leaf supports digestion where stress has slowed the system, especially around fat digestion and upper-abdominal discomfort.
It is helpful for sluggish digestion, nausea after eating, and "heavy" post-meal sensations.

Some benefits may be:
- Improved digestion
- More consistent bowel movements in some individuals.

## Why it helps under chronic stress.

Chronic stress reduces digestive secretions, bile flow, and enzyme activity.
Artichoke leaf increases bile production and movement, improving fat digestion and reducing pressure on the upper GI tract.

## Symptoms that may shift
- Sluggish/delayed digestion.

## Cross-system overlap
- Liver support (hepatoprotective antioxidant effects)
- Cholesterol-lowering activity in long-term trials.

## Clinician note.
- Generally, well tolerated

Use with care in:
- Bile duct obstruction
- Gallstone disease (avoid or supervise clinically)
- Pregnancy (limited data).

Mechanisms and findings:
- Cynarin + caffeoylquinic acids stimulate bile flow

- RCTs demonstrate improvement in dyspepsia symptoms
- Hepatoprotective effects via antioxidant mechanisms.

## References

Walker, A. F., et al. (2001). Artichoke leaf extract for dyspepsia. *Phytomedicine*, *8*(9), 709–714.

ESCOP Monographs: *Cynarae folium*.

Ben Salem, M., et al. (2015). Artichoke extract: hepatoprotective mechanisms. *Food & Function*, *6*(4), 1253–1261.

### *Ulmus rubra* (Slippery elm)

*(Primary actions: demulcent, mucilaginous, soothing to irritated mucosa)*

### What it does

Slippery elm coats and soothes irritated digestive tissue. It is particularly useful when stress has contributed to reflux, throat irritation from reflux episodes, or general upper gut sensitivity.

Some benefits may be:
- A soothing effect on the upper digestive tract
- Reduced irritation from reflux.

### Why it helps under chronic stress.

Stress increases gastric acid fluctuations and can heighten mucosal sensitivity. Slippery elm's mucilage forms a protective layer over irritated tissue, reducing discomfort while the system recalibrates.

## Symptoms that may shift

- Mild reflux
- Upper GI irritation.

## Cross-system overlap

- Mild bowel-regulating effects if the mucilage reaches the lower GI tract.

## Clinician note.

Generally well tolerated.

Considerations:
- Must be taken away from medications (can reduce absorption)
- Sustainability concerns - formulation choice should prioritise ethically sourced product
- Contraindications minimal.

Mechanisms and findings:
- Mucilage polysaccharides coat mucosa and reduce irritation
- Preliminary studies/formulations show symptom improvement in GERD-like patterns.

## References

Gao, L., et al. (2018). Review of demulcent herbs for upper GI irritation. *J Ethnopharmacol, 220*, 81–90.

ESCOP Monographs: *Ulmi cortex*.

## 15.6 - Pain and Inflammation Herbs

### Introduction

Long-term stress doesn't just drain your energy - it can turn up inflammatory signalling in the body. When the system is under prolonged pressure, inflammatory mediators increase, and for some people this shows up as pain, stiffness, tension, or flare-ups.

This section looks at the herbs with the strongest evidence for supporting healthy inflammatory responses. These are not quick fixes, and they're not substitutes for medical care, but they can play a role in helping the body settle when inflammation and stress have been working together for too long.

As always, it's important to work with a qualified health practitioner. They can tailor combinations, check interactions, and ensure the herbs chosen are appropriate for your situation.

### Why Stress Increases Inflammatory Mediators

Chronic stress activates the **HPA axis** and **sympathetic nervous system**, increasing cortisol and catecholamines. Over time, this can shift the immune system toward a pro-inflammatory state (McEwen & McEwen, 2017). Research shows prolonged stress is linked to increased levels of:

- Interleukin-6 (IL-6)
- C-reactive protein (CRP)
- Tumour necrosis factor-$\alpha$ (TNF-$\alpha$)

(Segerstrom & Miller, 2004; Rohleder, 2014).

## How Inflammation Drives Chronic Pain

Inflammation can sensitise nerve pathways involved in pain perception. Key mechanisms include:

- Increased prostaglandins (pain mediators)
- Sensitisation of nociceptors
- Changes in spinal cord pain processing pathways
- Muscle tension secondary to prolonged states of stress.

(Kim & Nabeshima, 2011; Vachon-Presseau, 2018).

## When Stress is Ongoing and Inflammatory Mediators Stay Elevated

When this is the case, some people experience:

- Worsening back or joint pain
- Muscle tightness
- Flare-ups of old injuries
- Generalised achiness.

Understanding this link helps explain why anti-inflammatory herbs, along with strong research support, can be useful during recovery.

### 1. *Curcuma longa* (Turmeric / Curcumin)

#### Primary actions

Anti-inflammatory, antioxidant, COX-2 modulation, NF-$\kappa$B inhibition.

#### What it does

Curcumin helps regulate inflammatory pathways commonly activated during long-term stress. Some benefits might include:

- Reduced stiffness
- Easing of joint or muscle discomfort
- Improved mobility
- Support for inflammatory balance.

**Why it helps in stress-related inflammatory states.**

Curcumin modulates inflammatory cytokines including IL-6 and TNF-α - the same mediators that rise under chronic stress exposure. It also influences oxidative pathways involved in pain perception.

**Symptoms that may shift**

- General inflammatory pain
- Joint discomfort
- Muscle aches
- Swelling or stiffness.

**Cross-system overlap**

- Gut anti-inflammatory support
- Mood and cognitive benefits in some trials.

**Clinician note.**

- Australian supplements carry a warning: *In very rare cases, Curcuma species may harm the liver. Stop use and see a doctor if you have yellowing skin/eyes or unusual: fatigue, nausea, appetite loss, abdominal pain, dark urine, or itching*
- Use with care in people taking anticoagulants.
- High doses may cause mild digestive upset.

**Key References**

Daily, J. W., et al. (2016). Efficacy of curcumin for osteoarthritis. *Journal of Medicinal Food, 19*(8), 717–729.

WHO Monographs: *Curcuma longa.*

ESCOP Monographs: *Curcumae longae rhizoma.*

## 2. *Boswellia serrata*

### Primary actions

5-LOX inhibition, anti-inflammatory, analgesic.

### What it does

Boswellia is well known for reducing inflammatory discomfort, especially where stiffness or swelling are present. Some benefits might include:

- Reduced joint pain
- Improved walking or movement comfort
- Decreased morning stiffness.

### Why it helps in stress-related inflammatory states.

Boswellia targets leukotriene pathways that become more active when stress increases systemic inflammation.

### Symptoms that may shift

- Osteoarthritic pain
- Inflammatory joint discomfort
- Movement-related pain.

### Cross-system overlap

- Gut inflammatory balance
- Respiratory inflammatory support.

**Clinician note.**

- Generally well-tolerated
- Use with care in individuals with reflux (may aggravate symptoms in some).

**Key References**

Kimmatkar, N., et al. (2003). Efficacy of *Boswellia serrata* in osteoarthritis. *Phytomedicine, 10*(1), 3–7.

Sengupta, K., et al. (2010). Boswellia extract for OA of knee. *Arthritis Research & Therapy, 12*(4), R153.

ESCOP Monographs: *Boswelliae serratae extractum*.

### 3. *Harpagophytum procumbens* (Devil's Claw)

**Primary actions**

Anti-inflammatory, analgesic, COX-2 modulation.

**What it does**

Often used for back pain, muscle discomfort, and joint stiffness. Some benefits might include:

- Improved mobility
- Reduced musculoskeletal pain
- Support for chronic lower back discomfort.

**Why it helps in stress-related inflammatory states.**

Devil's Claw influences inflammatory mediators that activate pain pathways under stress-related cytokine elevation.

## Symptoms that may shift

- Chronic back pain
- Joint pain
- Tension-related discomfort.

## Cross-system overlap

- Mild digestive support (bitters) in whole-root extracts.

## Clinician note.

- Well tolerated
- Avoid in gastric or duodenal ulcers (mild bitter effect)
- Use caution with anticoagulants.

## Key References

Gagnier, J. J., et al. (2004). Herbal medicine for low back pain: systematic review. *BMJ, 329,* 1377.

ESCOP Monographs: *Harpagophyti radix.*

## 4. *Salix alba* (White Willow Bark)

### Primary actions

Analgesic, anti-inflammatory (salicin → salicylic acid).

### What it does

Traditionally used for general musculoskeletal pain. Some benefits might include:

- Easing mild to moderate pain
- Support for osteoarthritis discomfort
- Reduced tension-related headache pain.

### Why it helps in stress-related inflammatory states.

Salicin supports inflammatory balance in pathways associated with stress-induced pain sensitisation.

### Symptoms that may shift

- Muscular aches
- Osteoarthritic pain
- Tension-type headaches.

### Cross-system overlap

- Mild fever support
- Anti-inflammatory support in generalised states.

### Clinician note.

- Avoid in salicylate sensitivity
- Use caution in people taking anticoagulants or antiplatelet medication
- Avoid in children, due to theoretical Reye's syndrome risk.

### Key References

Chrubasik, S., et al. (2000). White willow bark extract efficacy. *Phytomedicine, 7*(6), 417–424.

ESCOP Monographs: *Salicis cortex.*

### 5. *Zingiber officinale* (Ginger)

### Primary actions

Anti-inflammatory, analgesic, COX/LOX inhibition.

## What it does

Ginger supports inflammatory balance and may reduce pain in conditions involving muscle tension or joint discomfort. Some benefits might include:

- Reduced period pain
- Improved muscle comfort after strain
- Eased joint pain in some individuals.

## Why it helps in stress-related inflammatory states.

Ginger influences both cyclooxygenase and lipoxygenase pathways - mediators increased during chronic stress states.

## Symptoms that may shift

- Dysmenorrhoea pain
- Muscle soreness
- Inflammatory joint discomfort.

## Cross-system overlap

- Digestive support (carminative)
- Nausea support.

## Clinician note.

- Generally well tolerated
- Use caution with anticoagulants
- May cause reflux in some individuals.

## Key References

Black, C. D., et al. (2010). Ginger and muscle pain. *Journal of Pain*, *11*(9), 894–903.

Daily, J. W., et al. (2015). Ginger for OA: Meta-analysis. *Osteoarthritis & Cartilage, 23*, 363–371.

ESCOP Monographs: *Zingiberis rhizoma.*

## CHAPTER 15.7 - Other Supplements: A Special Mention

Not everything fits neatly into the "vitamin," "mineral," or "herbal" categories. Some supplements sit in their own lane - well researched, clinically useful, and often beneficial during stress recovery, but not tied to one body system alone.

This chapter offers clear, evidence-based explanations for a handful of nutrients that consistently show up in clinical practice and research. These aren't stand-alone treatments and they're certainly not required for everyone, but many people find them helpful during the recalibration phase.

As always:
**Please work with a qualified healthcare professional** before taking any of these.
They're not appropriate for every person or every condition, and a practitioner can assess interactions, safety, and your individual needs.

### 1. Coenzyme Q10 (CoQ10 / Ubiquinone / Ubiquinol)

#### What it does

CoQ10 is one of the body's primary antioxidants and a key part of mitochondrial energy production. Under chronic stress, oxidative load increases, and mitochondrial efficiency can take a hit. CoQ10 helps support steady energy production at a cellular level.

#### Some benefits might include:

- More stable day-to-day energy
- Reduced perception of fatigue
- Support during periods of physical or emotional depletion.

**Why it matters in stress recovery.**

Chronic stress increases oxidative stress markers (particularly in the mitochondria). CoQ10 supports mitochondrial function and may help restore energy balance.

**Symptoms that may shift**

- Fatigue
- Exertional tiredness
- Low stamina.

**Clinician note.**

Well tolerated

*Use with care alongside anticoagulants.
Ubiquinol may be preferable in older adults or those with impaired conversion.

**Key References**

Littarru, G. P., & Tiano, L. (2010). Clinical aspects of CoQ10: antioxidant and bioenergetic role. *Molecular Biotechnology, 37*, 31–37.

Hernández-Camacho, J. D., et al. (2018). Mitochondrial function & CoQ10. *Oxidative Medicine and Cellular Longevity, 2018*, 1–16.

## 2. Omega-3 Fatty Acids (EPA & DHA)

### What they do

Omega-3 fatty acids support inflammation balance, cell membrane function, brain health, and nervous system stability. They're among the most researched nutrients for mood, inflammation, and stress-related physiology.

### Some benefits might include:

- Improved cognitive clarity
- Support for mood stability
- Reduced inflammatory discomfort
- Support for cardiovascular health.

### Why they matter in stress recovery.

Long-term stress is associated with elevated inflammatory cytokines (IL-6, TNF-$\alpha$). EPA and DHA help regulate inflammatory signalling and support healthy neurotransmitter function.

### Symptoms that may shift

- Inflammatory pain
- Dry skin.

### Clinician note.

Use with care in people on anticoagulants.
Choose high-quality, low-oxidation products.

### Key References

Grosso, G., et al. (2014). Omega-3s and depression: systematic review. *PLoS One, 9*(5), e96905.

Calder, P. C. (2015). Omega-3s and inflammation. *Nutrients, 7*, 273–300.

### 3. Glutamine (L-Glutamine)

**What it does**

Glutamine is the primary fuel source for intestinal epithelial cells. During prolonged stress, digestive function can change, and the gut lining may become more vulnerable. Glutamine supports gut integrity and helps maintain a healthy mucosal barrier.

**Some benefits might include:**

- Reduced digestive discomfort
- Support for gut lining repair
- Improved tolerance to stress-related GI changes.

**Why it matters in stress recovery.**

Research shows that chronic stress affects intestinal permeability and mucosal health. Glutamine helps restore normal barrier function.

**Symptoms that may shift**

- Bloating
- Mild digestive irritation
- Discomfort linked with stress.

**Clinician note.**

- Well tolerated.
- Avoid in people with severe liver disease unless medically supervised (due to ammonia pathways).

**Key References**

Kim, M. H., & Kim, H. (2017). Role of glutamine in gut health. *Journal of the Korean Society for Applied Biological Chemistry, 60*(1), 1–5.

Zhou, Q., et al. (2020). Stress, gut permeability & glutamine. *Nutrients, 12*(11), 3338.

## 4. L-Theanine

*(Placed here, not in herbal medicine, because it is an amino acid, not a plant extract.)*

**What it does**

Theanine supports alpha-wave activity in the brain, associated with calm focus, rather than sedation. It helps modulate stress responses without reducing alertness.

**Some benefits might include:**

- Reduced mental tension
- Calmer cognitive processing
- Improved ability to focus.

**Why it matters in stress recovery.**

Theanine has been shown to reduce markers of acute psychological stress and assist with emotional regulation by modulating glutamate and GABA pathways.

**Clinician note.**

- Well tolerated.
- No major interactions documented at standard supplemental levels.

- Safe with most SSRIs based on current evidence.

**Key References**

Hidese, S., et al. (2019). Effects of L-theanine on stress-related symptoms. *Nutrients, 11*(10), 2362.

Juneja, L. R., et al. (1999). L-theanine and alpha-wave activity. *Trends in Food Science & Technology, 10*(6–7), 199–204.

## 5. Lactoferrin

### What it does

Lactoferrin is a naturally occurring iron-binding glycoprotein, with antimicrobial and immunomodulatory properties. It supports immune balance without overstimulation.

### Some benefits might include:

- Reduced frequency of minor infections.

### Why it matters in stress recovery.

Chronic stress affects immune signalling and increases susceptibility to mild infections. Lactoferrin helps modulate immune pathways associated with stress-induced immune shifts.

### Symptoms that may shift

- Frequent minor infections
- Immune vulnerability during or after stress
- Digestive discomfort (due to secondary GI benefits documented in some trials).

**Clinician note.**

- Use with care in individuals with milk protein allergy (as it is derived from dairy).
- Generally well tolerated.

**Key References**

Legrand, D. (2016). Lactoferrin: immune regulation. *Biochemistry and Cell Biology*, *94*(1), 26–30.

Ochoa, T. J., et al. (2015). Lactoferrin and host defence. *Journal of Applied Microbiology*, *119*, 1541–1551.

### 15.8 - Dietary Choices: Feeding Your Body

Nutrition plays a practical role in recovery from long-term stress. When the body has been under sustained pressure, several systems- digestion, immune function and energy regulation- may not operate as efficiently. Certain dietary patterns support these systems while they recalibrate. Others place additional load on processes that are already working harder than usual.

This chapter outlines evidence-based naturopathic dietary principles that support physical stability during recovery. These are not rules, and they are not prescriptive. They are simply guidelines that help the body function more efficiently.

#### 1. Foods and Substances to Reduce

The focus here is physiological impact, not judgement. These items increase metabolic, inflammatory, or neurological load in ways that can affect recovery.

## 1.1 Alcohol

Alcohol affects sleep quality, increases inflammatory signalling, and places additional strain on the liver. It can temporarily alter mood but often contributes to greater fatigue and disrupted sleep cycles.

Reducing intake can support more consistent energy and improved restorative sleep.

**Key evidence:**
Alcohol disrupts REM and slow-wave sleep and increases next-day fatigue (Roehrs & Roth, 2001).

## 1.2 Caffeine

Caffeine stimulates the central nervous system and increases catecholamine activity. This can be helpful for alertness but may worsen anxiety, palpitations, digestive discomfort, or sleep disruption in individuals recovering from chronic stress.

Reducing total intake, or timing it earlier in the day, can improve symptoms for some people.

**Key evidence:**
Caffeine increases sympathetic activation and can disrupt sleep latency and efficiency (Smith, 2002).

## 1.3 Ultra-processed foods, artificial additives, and preservatives

Highly processed foods often contain stabilisers, emulsifiers, preservatives, artificial sweeteners and colourings. These may contribute to gastrointestinal irritation and, in some individuals, altered microbiome composition.

Focusing on whole or minimally processed foods lowers the overall digestive and metabolic load.

**Key evidence:**
Emulsifiers and artificial sweeteners can alter gut microbial composition and increase intestinal permeability in susceptible individuals (Suez et al., 2014).

### 1.4 Fast food and packaged convenience foods

These products commonly contain high levels of salt, refined carbohydrates, poor-quality fats and additives. They tend to provide low micronutrient density, which is relevant when the body is replenishing nutrients affected by long-term stress.

Reducing frequency supports steadier digestion and energy.

## 2. Foods to Prioritise

These choices help deliver consistent nutrients, support digestion, and encourage better recovery of systems, disrupted by prolonged stress.

### 2.1 Fresh vegetables and fruits

A wide variety of vegetables and fruits provides:

- Vitamins and minerals
- Antioxidants
- Fibre
- Phytonutrients, which are important for immune and metabolic function.

Higher intake is consistently associated with improved physical and psychological wellbeing.

**Key evidence:**
Higher fruit and vegetable consumption correlates with improved mood and reduced inflammatory markers (Liu, 2013).

## 2.2 Whole grains

Whole grains provide fibre, B vitamins, and slow-release carbohydrates. This supports more even energy throughout the day and healthier digestive function.

Examples: Oats, brown rice, barley, quinoa, buckwheat.

## 2.3 Quality protein sources

Lean meats, poultry, eggs, legumes, dairy (if tolerated), and fish supply amino acids, required for neurotransmitter production, tissue repair, and immune function. Fish rich in omega-3 fatty acids also support inflammatory balance.

**Key evidence:**
Omega-3 intake is associated with reduced inflammation and improved mood regulation (Calder, 2015).

## 2.4 Avoid processed meats

Processed meats contain preservatives such as nitrites, along with high salt and saturated fat. They are consistently associated with increased inflammatory load.

Prioritising fresh, unprocessed protein reduces unnecessary metabolic strain.

## 2.5 Fresh vegetable juices

Fresh vegetable juices can supply concentrated micronutrients, particularly during times of reduced appetite or digestive fluctuation. They are not a substitute for whole vegetables, but can complement overall intake.

Selecting mostly vegetable-based juices helps avoid sharp increases in blood glucose.

## 3. A Practical Naturopathic Framework

These dietary choices support the systems most affected by chronic stress:

- **Digestive function** (fibre, reduced irritants)
- **Immune function** (phytonutrients, antioxidants)
- **Energy regulation** (whole foods over refined carbohydrates)
- **Inflammatory balance** (reduced alcohol, improved nutrient density).

This is not about strict dietary rules. It is about reducing unnecessary physical load and supplying nutrients that help the body recalibrate more efficiently.

## 15.9 - Movement and Lifestyle Fundamentals

Recovery after long-term stress or destabilising interpersonal environments is not achieved through dramatic lifestyle overhauls. The nervous system responds best to small, repeatable inputs. This chapter outlines evidence-based movement and lifestyle approaches that support recalibration, without pushing your system into further strain.

This is not a fitness chapter. It is a stability chapter.

The goal here is to help understand why certain practices are physiologically useful during recovery and how they can be applied at a pace that matches their current capacity.

## 1. Why Movement Matters in Recovery

Prolonged stress affects several systems simultaneously: the HPA axis, cardiovascular response, muscle tension patterns, sleep, and digestion. Light-to-moderate physical activity assists each of these systems in stabilising.

The aim is not intensity.
The aim is consistency.

**Evidence shows that:**

- Regular movement reduces baseline sympathetic activation
- Light aerobic activity supports improved sleep quality
- Walking increases vagal tone in some individuals
- Movement increases circulation of myokines that support mood regulation
- Physical activity reduces inflammatory markers associated with chronic stress.

These effects occur even at low doses - far below what is typically discussed in fitness literature.

**References:**
Hamer, M., & Steptoe, A. (2007); Wegner et al. (2014); Loprinzi et al. (2013).

## 2. Practical Movement Options (Evidence-Based)

This section outlines types of movement that have evidence for supporting stress recovery. None of these require high energy output or advanced fitness levels.

## 2.1 Walking

Walking is one of the most studied low-intensity activities for nervous system regulation.

Documented benefits include:

- Reduced perceived stress
- Improved sleep latency
- Increased cardiovascular variability (indicator of better stress tolerance)
- Improved cognitive processing after chronic stress exposure.

Even short, regular walks are beneficial.

**References:**
Merom et al. (2008); Teixeira et al. (2013).

## 2.2 Gentle Strength Work

Light resistance training has been shown to stabilise blood glucose, improve muscular tension patterns, and support more grounded physical awareness. This is relevant after long-term stress, where muscle tension is often chronic and involuntary.

Strength work does **not** need to involve heavy weights. Bodyweight movements and light resistance are sufficient.

**Reference:**
Strickland & Smith (2014).

## 2.3 Yoga (Evidence-Based)

Yoga is widely studied for stress modulation. Clinical evidence shows improvements in:

- Anxiety

- Autonomic nervous system balance
- Mild to moderate depressive symptoms
- Sleep quality
- Cortisol regulation in some studies.

Gentle, non-heated yoga is generally the most supportive during recovery, as high-intensity forms may elevate stress hormones.

**References:**
Field (2011); Pascoe et al. (2017).

### 2.4 Stretching and Mobility Work

Basic stretching reduces muscle tension, particularly in the shoulders, neck, and lower back -common areas affected by prolonged stress. Mobility work supports a calmer physical baseline, by reducing the level of chronic contraction held in the musculature.

**Reference:**
Afonso et al. (2021).

### 2.5 Nature Exposure (Green Exercise)

Spending time outdoors, especially in green or blue spaces, is associated with:

- Reduced sympathetic activation
- Lower rumination
- Lower physiological arousal
- Improved working memory
- Reduced cortisol in some individuals.

This can include walking, sitting outside, gardening, or light movement.

**References:**
Bratman et al. (2015); Twohig-Benett & Jones (2018).

## 3. Supporting Lifestyle Practices

Lifestyle change in recovery centres around predictable, low-stress routines that assist physical stability.

### 3.1 Regularity of sleep and waking times

The nervous system responds well to predictability. Regular waking and sleep times support circadian rhythm restoration, which can be disrupted during periods of chronic stress.

**Reference:**
Walker (2017).

### 3.2 Morning light exposure

Exposure to natural light in the morning helps regulate circadian rhythm, supports cortisol awakening response, and improves sleep quality later in the evening.

**References:**
Khalsa et al. (2003).

### 3.3 Reduced sensory load

Stress can heighten sensory sensitivity. Lowering background stimulation - noise, clutter, competing demands - gives the nervous system space to downshift.

### 3.4 Social contact that is predictable and low-pressure

Positive interpersonal interactions support recovery, but only when they are:

- Non-demanding

- Predictable
- Non-critical
- Emotionally safe.

Evidence shows that supportive social connection reduces the physiological burden of stress and lowers inflammatory signalling.

**Reference:**
Uchino (2006).

Movement and lifestyle support do not need to be dramatic to be effective.

Small, repeatable steps produce better outcomes than strenuous bursts of effort, particularly during recovery.

## 15.10 - Environmental Stabilisation (Your Home as a Healing Space)

When the nervous system has been running on chronic activation for a long time, the environment you live in plays a measurable role in how easily your body stabilises. This chapter outlines what an evidence-informed, calm-supportive home environment looks like, without turning your space into a project or implying you need a perfect aesthetic.

### 1. Why Your Environment Matters in Recovery

Environments influence stress physiology more than most people realise. Research shows that:

- Clutter increases cognitive load
- Loud, unpredictable noise increases sympathetic activation

- Low lighting, fresh air and natural elements, can support calmer baseline states
- Predictable environments reduce the need for constant monitoring
- A sense of control over your space reduces perceived stress.

These effects are subtle, but cumulative. A steady, low-demand environment gives your nervous system fewer signals to interpret as potential threat.

**References:**
Evans & Wener (2007); Kaplan (1995); Korpela et al. (2018).

## 2. Predictability: The Foundation of Environmental Stabilisation

After prolonged stress, the nervous system responds well to predictable cues.
Your home does not need to be pristine - it simply needs to be *legible*.

### Environmental predictability can include:

- Knowing where things are
- Reducing unnecessary visual stimulation
- Maintaining small, consistent routines (e.g. dishes done, laundry in one spot)
- Creating "low-demand" areas, where nothing needs to be done.

Predictability reduces the number of decisions you make each day, which supports cognitive recovery after prolonged stress.

**Reference:**
Vohs et al. (2014).

## 3. Light, Air, and Sensory Load

These are the basics that support physiological downshifting.

### 3.1 Light

Natural light exposure supports circadian rhythm regulation. Brighter daytime light and dimmer evening light helps stabilise sleep–wake patterns.

If natural light is limited, consistent artificial lighting can be used - the key is regularity.

**Reference:**
Khalsa et al. (2003).

### 3.2 Air

Fresh air improves perceived mental clarity and reduces symptoms associated with indoor pollutants. Opening a window daily supports ventilation, which can help individuals who experience fatigue or low mood after long-term stress.

**Reference:**
Allen et al. (2016).

### 3.3 Sensory Load

High sensory input (noise, clutter, flashing screens, strong odours) places continuous demands on the stress response system.
Reducing sensory load is not about "minimalism" - it's about lowering background activation.

Helpful adjustments can include:

- Reducing noise where possible
- Keeping certain areas visually simple

- Choosing calmer colour palettes
- Limiting competing stimuli in sleep and rest areas.

These changes do not need to be aesthetic. They need to be *functional*.

## 4. Creating Micro-Zones of Support

You do not need a full home overhaul.
A few dedicated "stable" spaces can be enough.

### 4.1 A Calm Corner

This might be:

- A chair near a window
- A space with a lamp and comfortable blanket
- A quiet area where you can read, breathe, or sit without expectation.

Function: A consistent, low-demand micro-environment, where your nervous system learns that nothing is required of it.

### 4.2 A Sleep-Protective Zone

Your sleep environment benefits from fewer stimuli and predictable cues.

Evidence-based elements include:

- Darker room
- Stable temperature
- Limited noise
- Consistent bedtime lighting
- Reduced screens in the hour before sleep.

This is not about strict rules; it's about reducing barriers to physiological rest.

**Reference:**
Walker (2017).

### 4.3 A Clarity Zone

This is a practical space where you can do tasks without competing distractions.
It helps with cognitive reorganisation after prolonged stress.

This could be a clear table, a quiet corner, or a desk with minimal items.

The purpose: Reduce cognitive load and support executive functioning, while it recalibrates.

## 5. Natural Elements

Exposure to natural elements, even indoors, can have measurable effects on stress physiology.

Evidence supports:

- Indoor plants reducing perceived stress and improving attention
- Views of nature lowering sympathetic activation
- Natural textures and colours improving perceived calm.

This is not about aesthetics or trends, it is about giving your nervous system environments it recognises as non-threatening.

**References:**
Bringslimark et al. (2009); Berto (2014).

## 6. Reducing Environmental Triggers

Long-term stress often heightens reactivity to environmental cues.

Common triggers may include:

- Sudden noises
- Unexpected visual clutter
- Reminders of past environments
- Overstimulating media
- Chaotic spaces.

Making small adjustments can lower baseline activation and give the nervous system space to stabilise.

You do not need a perfect home to recover.

A calm environment is not a luxury, it's simply another tool.

Your home environment does not need to look magazine-ready to be effective.

## 15.11 Building Predictable Routines

When the nervous system has been exposed to chronic stress, inconsistency, or unpredictability, even small daily tasks can feel disorganised or fragmented. Predictable routines help rebuild internal order by reducing decision-making load and giving the stress response system fewer variables to manage.

This is not about discipline or perfection.
It is about giving your body and mind a stable framework to work within, so they don't have to continually scan, adjust, or compensate.

## Why Predictability Matters

Research across stress physiology and cognitive science shows:

- Predictable routines reduce perceived stress
- Habits reduce cognitive load and decision fatigue
- Consistency supports executive functioning
- Steady patterns help stabilise sleep–wake cycles
- Routine-oriented environments reduce sympathetic activation.

Predictability helps the system shift away from chronic readiness. This is particularly useful after long periods of relational instability, where patterns have been inconsistent or confusing.

## References:
Diamond (2013); McEwen & McEwen (2017); Galla & Duckworth (2015).

## 2. Routine as a Biological Cue

A predictable routine gives the nervous system repeated signals that:

- Nothing sudden is happening
- There is time to complete a task
- The environment is not demanding constant vigilance
- The day has structure.

These signals help recalibrate the HPA axis and support autonomic balance.

A routine is not about productivity, it's about lowering the system's baseline activation.

### 3. Start Small: Micro-Routines

Full routines can feel overwhelming early in recovery. Micro-routines are small actions repeated daily or weekly, that don't require significant planning.

Examples include:

- Starting the day with the same simple action (e.g. opening a blind)
- Having one consistent mealtime
- Placing keys or essentials in the same location
- A set time to walk, stretch, or check in with your body
- Winding down at the same general time each evening.

These are not performance-based, they simply give your system predictable anchors.

### 4. Why Routines Feel Different After Stress

Chronic stress affects:

- Executive functioning (planning, sequencing, decision-making)
- Working memory
- Energy regulation
- Sleep patterns
- Motivation pathways.

This means routines may feel harder to initiate at first. This is not a lack of willpower, it is a temporary neurobiological effect that improves with consistency and time.

**References:**
Arnsten (2009); LeDoux (2012).

## 5. The Role of External Supports

External structure compensates for internal fatigue.

These supports may include:

- Reminders
- Visual cues
- Simple checklists
- Calendars
- Dedicated spaces for specific tasks
- These tools help reduce the number of decisions your prefrontal cortex must make during the day.

Using supports is not a sign of struggling, it is a sign of recalibration.

## 6. Anchor Points: The Non-Negotiable Few

Anchor points are core routines that help regulate biological rhythm.

These might include:

- Consistent waking time
- Regular meals
- A wind-down period before bed
- Some form of movement
- A brief moment of stillness or quiet.

These anchors support endocrine stability, digestion and circadian rhythm, more than most people recognise.

**References:**
Khalsa et al. (2003); Walker (2017).

Routines don't need to be aspirational.
They don't need to look productive or impressive.

A routine is not a self-improvement project.
It's simply a predictable rhythm that helps your system downshift.

If your "routine" is that you have the same cup of tea every morning, at roughly the same time, that counts too.

The routine I began while I was rebuilding was to make a cup of tea when I woke up in the morning, grab my journal, and take it outside. As I drink my cup of tea, I write anything and everything, and I still do it every day. It's my anchor and I got this idea from a book called "The Artist's Way" by Julia Cameron. It's worked for me and sets me up for the day.

# CHAPTER SIXTEEN

# Pulling it All Together With the Hogan Method

I've developed the Hogan method to walk through the information, so that you can find your way back to the shining light that is you.

The Hogan Method is not a shortcut.
It's not a cure.
It's not a replacement for therapy.
It is a structured way to support the body and mind in returning to equilibrium after prolonged stress or destabilising relationships.

It works alongside any trauma-informed psychological care, not instead of it.

## 1. The Hogan Method Approach

The Hogan Method is a whole-body approach I developed over many years working with clients who presented with:

- Chronic stress
- Nervous system dysregulation
- Post-relationship destabilisation
- Digestive disturbances
- Sleep disruption
- Fatigue
- Pain or inflammatory flare-ups
- Nutrient depletion from long-term stress
- Burn out

Most of my clients functioned well on the outside. Most were exhausted on the inside.

The Hogan Method brings together the core elements we've covered in this book:

1. Understanding what has happened (clarity + education).
2. Stabilising the body first (nervous system, digestion, sleep, immunity).
3. Reintroducing nutritional and herbal support (evidence-based).
4. Building predictability (routines, rhythms, anchoring).
5. Supporting the system as it recalibrates.
6. Reconnecting with your baseline gradually.

It's a model, not a mandate.

## 2. What the Hogan Method Is Not

This is important to be explicit about.

However, this Hogan Method does **not**:

- Diagnose narcissism
- Pathologise people
- Provide psychological treatment
- Prescribe medication
- Promise transformation
- Involve cognitive processing of trauma
- Replace trauma-informed therapeutic care.

The Method supports the **physiology,** so the rest of your recovery has a stable foundation.

## 3. Why the Method Works in Stages

Recovery from prolonged relational stress is not linear. The body recalibrates in different ways, at different times.

### 3.1 Safety recognition

The nervous system registers reduced external threat.

### 3.2 Physiological stabilisation

Breathing, sleep, digestion and cortisol regulate incrementally.

### 3.3 Nutrient restoration

Deficiencies created by chronic activation begin to normalise.

### 3.4 Energy return

Small pockets of capacity reappear.

### 3.5 Cognitive clarity

Micro-cognition, memory and executive function improve.

### 3.6 Emotional differentiation

Feelings stop clustering and become more organised.

The Hogan Method aligns with this natural sequence - it does not force anything outside your system's current capacity.

## 4. Core Pillars of the Hogan Method

### Pillar 1 - Clarity Through Education

People stabilise faster when they understand what has happened. This book forms that foundation.

### Pillar 2 - Nervous System Support

Breath patterns, micro-routines, evidence-supported nutrients and herbs, help regulate autonomic tone.

### Pillar 3 - Digestive and Immune Restoration

Chronic stress affects the gut–brain axis, immune signalling, motility and nutrient absorption. This is addressed systematically.

### Pillar 4 - Sleep Recalibration

Sleep quality improves gradually with structure, nutrients, herbal options and basic sleep hygiene.

### Pillar 5 - Inflammation and Pain Support

Long-term stress can elevate inflammatory mediators. Turmeric, Boswellia, Devil's claw, ginger and other evidence-based interventions support this stage.

### Pillar 6 - Thoughtful Supplementation

CoQ10, Omega-3, Lactoferrin, theanine, glutamine and others form the "special mentions" chapter for personalised care.

### Pillar 7 - Lifestyle Anchors

Movement, light exposure, predictable meals, hydration, environmental support, and daily anchors reduce load on the stress system.

**Pillar 8 - Reconnection With Self**

As physiological stability returns, people can identify preferences, boundaries and needs again - without internal noise drowning them out.

## 5. When to Seek Professional Support

This Method is designed to sit *beside* qualified care and I encourage you to seek a trauma-informed psychologist:

- A specialised narcissistic abuse therapy clinician
- A registered naturopath, nutritionist, herbalist, or integrative GP, who has a solid understanding of narcissistic traits
- Clinical assessment if symptoms persist or worsen.

Certain situations require specialised support:

- Financial, cultural or familial barriers to leaving
- Active coercive control
- Safety concerns
- Complex trauma symptoms
- Medical conditions that need supervision.

No book, including this one, replaces individualised care.

## 6. Where You Go From Here

Recovery is not a dramatic turning point.
It is a slow increase in capacity.

What you may notice:

- Steadier mornings
- Clearer thinking

- Decreased startle responses
- Improved digestion
- Fewer inflammatory flares
- Better sleep
- The ability to take a full breath
- Small decisions feeling less overwhelming.

These are the signs that the system is stabilising. This is where the Hogan Method is most effective - not at the crisis point, but at the point where recalibration has space to occur.

You do not need to implement everything at once. You are not behind if you take this slowly. Healing from long-term relational stress is complex, and your system will take the lead if you allow it.

### 7. A Final Note from Me

I wrote this book because I remember what it was like to stand where you are now knowing something was wrong, feeling the consequences in my body, but without a clear map for what came next. No compass. Just symptoms, confusion, and a nervous system doing its best to survive.

This was never about telling you to move on, reframe faster, or override what your body learned under pressure. It was about giving language to what you lived through, and physiology to what you felt - so the experience could finally make sense, without shame or judgement.

Your body has been keeping the score long before you had words for it. That wasn't failure. It was intelligence.

You are not behind.
You are not broken.

Your system adapted in the only ways it could to stay functional and safe.

If this book has done its job, you now have something I didn't have at the beginning: orientation. Enough clarity to trust what your body has been telling you, and enough understanding to begin choosing your way forward deliberately.

I've walked this terrain myself. I know how disorienting it can be. You don't need to rush, and you don't need to get it perfect. You just need a direction and the knowledge that your body can come with you.

That is what this work, and The Hogan Method, is here to support.

# CHAPTER REFERENCES

## Chapters 1, 2, and 3

Bowlby, J. (1988). *A secure base: Parent-child attachment and healthy human development.* Basic Books.

Cicchetti, D., & Toth, S. L. (2016). Child maltreatment and developmental psychopathology. *Child Development,* 87(2), 442–448.

Fisher, J. (2021). *Transforming the living legacy of trauma: A workbook for survivors and therapists.* PESI Publishing.

Gunnar, M. R., & Quevedo, K. (2007). The neurobiology of stress and development. *Annual Review of Psychology,* 58, 145–173.

Hinojosa, A. S., Gardner, W. L., Walker, H. J., Cogliser, C., & Gullifor, D. (2017). A review of cognitive dissonance theory in management research: Opportunities for further development. *Journal of Management,* 43(1), 170–199. https://doi.org/10.1177/0149206316668236

Linehan, M. M. (1993). *Skills training manual for treating borderline personality disorder.* Guilford Press. (Referenced solely for emotional invalidation research; no diagnostic usage.)

McEwen, B. S. (2007). Physiology and neurobiology of stress and adaptation: Central role of the brain. *Physiological Reviews,* 87(3), 873–904.

McEwen, B. S. (2022). Neurobiological and systemic effects of chronic stress. *Dialogues in Clinical Neuroscience,* 24(1), 1–12. https://doi.org/10.31887/DCNS.2022.24.1

Perry, B. D., & Szalavitz, M. (2017). *The boy who was raised as a dog.* Basic Books.

Porges, S. W. (2011). *The polyvagal theory.* W. W. Norton.

Porges, S. W. (2022). *Polyvagal safety: Attachment, communication, self-regulation.* W. W. Norton & Company.

Schore, A. N. (2001). Effects of early relational trauma on right brain development. *Infant Mental Health Journal,* 22(1–2), 201–269.

Walker, P. (2013). *Complex PTSD: From surviving to thriving.* Azure Coyote Publishing.

## Trauma Physiology and Nervous System

Porges, S. W. (2022). *Polyvagal Safety: Attachment, Communication, SelfRegulation.* New York: W. W. Norton.

Fisher, J. (2021). *Healing the Fragmented Selves of Trauma Survivors.* London: Routledge.

van der Kolk, B. (2014). *The Body Keeps the Score.* New York: Viking.

Payne, P., Levine, P. A., & CraneGodreau, M. A. (2015). Somatic experiencing and interoception. *Frontiers in Psychology,* 6, 93.

## Stress, Allostatic Load and Health

McEwen, B. S., & Akil, H. (2020). Revisiting the stress concept. *Journal of Neuroscience,* 40(1), 12–21.

McEwen, B. S. (2022). *The End of Stress as We Know It.* Washington, DC: Dana Press.

Thayer, J. F., & Lane, R. D. (2009). Neurovisceral integration. *Neuroscience & Biobehavioral Reviews,* 33(2), 81–88.

## Coercive Control and Relational Threat

Stark, E. (2007). *Coercive Control: The Entrapment of Women in Personal Life*. New York: Oxford University Press.

Dutton, D. G. (2007). *The Abusive Personality: Violence and Control in Intimate Relationships*. New York: Guilford Press.

Hinojosa, M. S., et al. (2017). Intimate partner violence and cognitive dissonance. *Journal of Family Violence*, 32, 637–648.

## Survival Strategies and Appeasement

Walker, P. (2013). *Complex PTSD: From Surviving to Thriving*. California: Azure Coyote.

Schore, A. N. (2019). *Right Brain Psychotherapy*. New York: W. W. Norton.

## Post-Separation Dynamics

Bancroft, L., & Silverman, J. G. (2002). *The Batterer as Parent: Addressing the Impact of Domestic Violence on Family Dynamics*. Thousand Oaks: Sage Publications.

Crossman, K. A., et al. (2016). Coercive control and post-separation abuse. *Partner Abuse*, 7(2), 161–183.

## Chapter 4 References

Fisher, J. (2021). *Transforming the living legacy of trauma: A workbook for survivors and therapists*. PESI Publishing.

Fitzcharles, M.-A., Cohen, S. P., & Clauw, D. J. (2021). Chronic primary pain: A review of mechanistic studies. *The Lancet*, 397(10289), 1762–1772.

Hinojosa, A. S., Gardner, W. L., Walker, H. J., Cogliser, C., & Gullifor, D. (2017). A review of cognitive dissonance theory in management research: Opportunities for further development. *Journal of Management*, 43(1), 170–199. https://doi.org/10.1177/0149206316668236

LeDoux, J. (2012). Rethinking the emotional brain. *Neuron*, 73(4), 653–676. https://doi.org/10.1016/j.neuron.2012.02.004

LeDoux, J. (2015). *Anxious: Using the Brain to Understand and Treat Fear and Anxiety*. Viking.

McEwen, B. S., & Wingfield, J. C. (2003). The concept of allostasis in biology and biomedicine. *Hormones and Behavior*, 43(1), 2–15.

Porges, S. W. (2011). *The polyvagal theory: Neurophysiological foundations of emotions, attachment, communication, and self-regulation*. W. W. Norton.

Segerstrom, S. C., & Miller, G. E. (2004). Psychological stress and the human immune system: A meta-analytic study of 30 years of inquiry. *Psychological Bulletin*, 130(4), 601–630.

van der Kolk, B. A. (2014). *The body keeps the score: Brain, mind, and body in the healing of trauma*. Viking.

## Chapter 5 References

Apkarian, A. V., Hashmi, J. A., & Baliki, M. N. (2011). Pain and the brain: Specificity and plasticity of the brain in clinical chronic pain. *Pain*, 152(3 Suppl), S49–S64.

Fitzcharles, M.-A., Cohen, S. P., & Clauw, D. J. (2021). Chronic primary pain: A review of mechanistic studies. *The Lancet*, 397(10289), 1762–1772.

McEwen, B. S., & Wingfield, J. C. (2003). The concept of allostasis in biology and biomedicine. *Hormones and Behavior, 43*(1), 2–15.

Porges, S. W. (2011). *The polyvagal theory: Neurophysiological foundations of emotions, attachment, communication, and self-regulation.* W. W. Norton.

Segerstrom, S. C., & Miller, G. E. (2004). Psychological stress and the human immune system: A meta-analytic study of 30 years of inquiry. *Psychological Bulletin, 130*(4), 601–630.

**Chapter 6 References**

Arnsten, A. F. T. (2009). Stress signalling pathways that impair prefrontal cortex structure and function. *Nature Reviews Neuroscience, 10*(6), 410–422.

Fisher, J. (2021). *Transforming the living legacy of trauma: A workbook for survivors and therapists.* Routledge.

LeDoux, J. (2015). *Anxious: Using the brain to understand and treat fear and anxiety.* Viking.

McEwen, B. S., & Wingfield, J. C. (2003). The concept of allostasis in biology and biomedicine. *Hormones and Behavior, 43*(1), 2–15.

Porges, S. W. (2011). *The polyvagal theory: Neurophysiological foundations of emotions, attachment, communication, and self-regulation.* W. W. Norton.

**Chapter 7 References**

Fisher, J. (2021). *Transforming the living legacy of trauma: A workbook for survivors and therapists.* PESI Publishing.

McEwen, B. S. (2007). Physiology and neurobiology of stress and adaptation: Central role of the brain. *Physiological Reviews, 87*(3), 873–904. https://doi.org/10.1152/physrev.00041.2006

Porges, S. W. (2004). Neuroception: A subconscious system for detecting threats and safety. *Zero to Three, 24*(5), 19–24.

Porges, S. W. (2011). *The polyvagal theory: Neurophysiological foundations of emotions, attachment, communication, and self-regulation.* W. W. Norton.

Tedeschi, R. G., & Calhoun, L. G. (2004). Posttraumatic growth: Conceptual foundations and empirical evidence. *Psychological Inquiry, 15*(1), 1–18. https://doi.org/10.1207/s15327965pli1501_01

van der Kolk, B. A. (2014). *The body keeps the score: Brain, mind, and body in the healing of trauma.* Viking.

## Chapter 8 – no references listed.

## Chapter 9 References

Arnsten, A. F. T. (2009). Stress signalling pathways that impair prefrontal cortex structure and function. *Nature Reviews Neuroscience, 10*(6), 410–422.

Bowen, M. (1978). *Family therapy in clinical practice.* Jason Aronson.

Campbell, W. K., & Miller, J. D. (2011). *The handbook of narcissism and narcissistic personality disorder: Theoretical approaches, empirical findings, and treatments.* Wiley.

Carnell, L., et al. (2020). Intermittent reinforcement and attachment vulnerability. *Journal of Social and Personal Relationships, 37*(5), 1334–1353.

Darke 2025 interdisciplinary reviewSpringerLink

Darke 2025 gaslighting and memoryTaylor & Francis Online

Durvasula, R. (2021). *Should I stay or should I go? Surviving a narcissistic relationship.* Post Hill Press.

Dutton, M. A., & Goodman, L. A. (2005). Coercion in intimate partner violence: Toward a new conceptualization. *Sex Roles, 52*(11–12), 743–756.

Fisher, H. (2017). The role of dopamine in romantic attraction. *Philosophical Transactions of the Royal Society B,* 372(1711).

Fisher, J. (2021). *Transforming the living legacy of trauma: A workbook for survivors and therapists.* PESI Publishing.

Freyd, J., & Smidt, A. (2019). DARVO: Deny, Attack, and Reverse Victim and Offender. *Journal of Trauma & Dissociation,* 20(3), 289–300.

Gottman, J. (2011). *The science of trust: Emotional attunement for couples.* Norton.

Herman, J. (2015). *Trauma and recovery.* Basic Books. (Original work published 1992)

Johnson, S. (2019). *Hold me tight.* Little, Brown Spark.

Klein 2023 qualitative analysis of gaslighting in romantic relationshipsWiley Online Library

Klein, Wood & Bartz 2025 theoretical framework for gaslightingSuzanne Wood, PhD

LeDoux, J. (2012). Rethinking the emotional brain. *Neuron, 73*(4), 653–676.

McEwen, B. (2007). Stress, adaptation, and allostasis. *Physiology Review*, 87(3), 873–904.

Mento 2023 on psychological violence and gaslighting in couplesscholar

Mikulincer, M., & Shaver, P. R. (2007). *Attachment in adulthood*. Guilford Press.

Minuchin, S. (1974). *Families and family therapy*. Harvard University Press.

Ogden, P., Minton, K., & Pain, C. (2006). *Trauma and the body: A sensorimotor approach to psychotherapy*. W.W. Norton.

Porges, S. (2011). *The polyvagal theory*. Norton.

Ronningstam, E. (2016). Pathological narcissism. In Livesley, J. W., Dimaggio, G., & Clarkin, J. F. (Eds.), *Integrated treatment for personality disorder* (pp. 133–146). Guilford Press.

Siegel, D. J. (1999). *The developing mind*. Guilford Press.

Stark, E. (2007). *Coercive control: How men entrap women in personal life*. Oxford University Press.

Strutzenberg, C., & Whisman, M. A. (2021). Early-stage romantic intensity and psychological distress. *Journal of Social and Clinical Psychology*, 40(2), 97–119.

Sweet, P. (2019). The sociology of gaslighting. *American Sociological Review*, 84(5), 851–875.

van der Kolk, B. (2014). *The body keeps the score*. Viking.

Day et al. 2025 – pathological narcissism significantly associated with coercive controlPMC

Fitz-Gibbon et al. 2024 – survivors' experiences of coercive control (Australia)Australian Institute of Criminology

AIHW & AIFS summaries of coercive control patterns (AU context)AIHW

**Grandiose Narcissism References**

American Psychiatric Association. (2022). *Diagnostic and Statistical Manual of Mental Disorders* (5th ed., text rev.).

Campbell, W. K., & Miller, J. D. (2011). *The handbook of narcissism and narcissistic personality disorder: Theoretical approaches, empirical findings, and treatments.* Wiley.

Ronningstam, E. (2016). Narcissistic personality disorder: Recognition and treatment. *The Journal of Psychotherapy Integration*, 26(2), 167–178.

**Covert (vulnerable) Narcissism References**

American Psychiatric Association. (2022). *Diagnostic and Statistical Manual of Mental Disorders* (5th ed., text rev.).

Dickinson, K. A., & Pincus, A. L. (2003). Interpersonal analysis of grandiose and vulnerable narcissism. *Journal of Personality Disorders*, 17(3), 188–207.

Kealy, D., & Ogrodniczuk, J. S. (2011). Vulnerable narcissism: The dark side of shame and attachment. *Journal of Psychiatric Practice*, 17(2), 89–99.

Pincus, A. L., & Lukowitsky, M. R. (2010). Pathological narcissism and narcissistic personality disorder. *Annual Review of Clinical Psychology*, 6, 421–446.

Baskin-Sommers et al. 2014 – empathy in NPDPMC

Simard et al. 2023 – meta-analysis on narcissism and empathyScienceDirect

di Giacomo et al. 2023 – "dark side of empathy" in NPDFrontiers

Ronningstam – clinical work on pathological narcissism/empathic functioningPsychiatry+1

Weinberg 2022 – current review of NPD, including empathy profiles

Mahadevan 2024 – interpersonal profiles of grandiose vs vulnerable narcissismWiley Online Library

Edershile et al. 2020 – fluctuations between grandiose and vulnerable statesPMC

Loeffler et al. 2020 – grandiose vs vulnerable in social anxiety context (helps explain "wobbly" socially)Frontiers

Weinberg 2022 – updated clinical view of pathological narcissism / NPDpsychiatryonline.org

## Communal (Benevolent) Narcissism References

American Psychiatric Association. (2022). *Diagnostic and Statistical Manual of Mental Disorders* (5th ed., text rev.).

Gebauer, J. E., Sedikides, C., Verplanken, B., & Maio, G. R. (2012). Communal narcissism. *Journal of Personality and Social Psychology*, 103(5), 854–878.

Nehrlich, A. D., Gebauer, J. E., Sedikides, C., & Abele, A. E. (2019). Communal narcissists' self-views: Evidence for positive illusions. *European Journal of Personality*, 33(2), 204–221.

## Malignant Narcissism Pattern References

The behavioural patterns described in this section are supported by peer-reviewed research across psychology, interpersonal violence, and coercive control literature. These sources describe **patterns of behaviour**, not diagnoses.

### Core Narcissistic and Malignant Behaviour Research

Miller, J. D., Campbell, W. K., & Pilkonis, P. A. (2010). *Narcissistic personality disorder: Relations with distress and functional impairment.* Journal of Personality Disorders, 24(5), 590–606.

Ronningstam, E. (2016). *Pathological narcissism and narcissistic personality disorder: Recent advances.* Current Psychiatry Reports, 18(9), 86.

Paulhus, D. L., & Williams, K. M. (2002). *The Dark Triad of personality.* Journal of Research in Personality, 36(6), 556–563.

### Aggression, Humiliation, and Exploitation

Reidy, D. E., Zeichner, A., Foster, J. D., & Martinez, M. A. (2008). *Effects of narcissistic entitlement and exploitativeness on human physical aggression.* Journal of Research in Personality, 42(6), 1492–1500.

Follingstad, D. R., Rutledge, L. L., Berg, B. J., Hause, E. S., & Polek, D. S. (1990). *The role of emotional abuse in physically abusive relationships.* Journal of Family Violence, 5(2), 107–120.

### Coercive Control and Punitive Behaviour

Stark, E. (2007). *Coercive control: How men entrap women in personal life.* Oxford University Press.

MacDonald, F. (2020). *Exploring coercive control in Australia.* Australian Journal of Family Law, 34, 1–22.

Fitz-Gibbon, K., McCulloch, J., & Maher, J. (2024). *Coercive control and criminalisation*. Palgrave Macmillan.

Australian Institute of Health and Welfare. (2022). *Family, domestic and sexual violence in Australia*. AIHW.

## Emerging Links Between Narcissism and Coercive Control

Day, A., Bowen, E., & Hollin, C. (2025). *Personality pathology and coercive control behaviours in intimate relationships*. (In press / emerging research cited conservatively).

## Nervous System, Trauma, and Long-Term Impact

Herman, J. L. (2015). *Trauma and recovery* (Updated ed.). Basic Books.

van der Kolk, B. A. (2014). *The body keeps the score*. Viking.

Porges, S. W. (2011). *The polyvagal theory*. W. W. Norton & Company.

## Chapter 10 References

Campbell, W. K., & Miller, J. D. (2011). The handbook of narcissism and narcissistic personality disorder: Theoretical approaches, empirical findings, and treatments. Wiley.

Durvasula, R. (2021). *"It's not you: Identifying narcissistic behaviors in relationships."*
(YouTube lectures, interviews, and published works on narcissistic relational dynamics.)

Ferster, C. B., & Skinner, B. F. (1957). *Schedules of reinforcement*. Appleton-Century-Crofts.

Freyd, J. J. (1997). Violations of power, adaptive blindness, and betrayal trauma theory. *Feminism & Psychology, 7*(1), 22–32.

Hinojosa, A. S., Gardner, W. L., Walker, H. J., Cogliser, C. C., & Gullifor, D. (2017). A review of cognitive dissonance theory in management research. *Journal of Management, 43*(1), 170–199.

Pincus, A. L., Cain, N. M., & Wright, A. G. (2009). Narcissistic grandiosity and narcissistic vulnerability. *Personality and Social Psychology Bulletin, 35*(10), 1323–1336.

Porges, S. W. (2011). *The polyvagal theory: Neurophysiological foundations of emotions, attachment, communication, and self-regulation.* Norton.

Ronningstam, E. (2016). *Pathological narcissism and narcissistic personality disorder in Axis I disorders.* American Psychiatric Publishing.

Streep, P. (2019). *Mastering manipulative relationships: Recognizing harmful patterns.* HarperCollins.

Sweet, P. L. (2019). The sociology of gaslighting. *American Sociological Review, 84*(5), 851–875.

## Chapter 11 References

Arnsten, A. F. (2009). Stress signalling pathways that impair prefrontal cortex structure and function. *Nature Reviews Neuroscience, 10*(6), 410–422.

Barrett, L. F. (2017). *How emotions are made: The secret life of the brain.* Houghton Mifflin Harcourt.

Caine, J., et al. (2020). Stress-related neuroendocrine responses and relational disruption. *Journal of Affective Disorders, 276*, 732–740.

Fisher, J. (2021). *Transforming the living legacy of trauma.* PESI Publishing.

Hinojosa, A. S., Gardner, W. L., Walker, H. J., Cogliser, C. C., & Gullifor, D. (2017). A review of cognitive dissonance theory in management research. *Journal of Management, 43*(1), 170–199.

LeDoux, J. (2020). *The deep history of ourselves: The four-billion-year story of how we got conscious brains.* Penguin.

McEwen, B. S. (2007). Physiology and neurobiology of stress and adaptation: central role of the brain. *Physiological Reviews, 87*(3), 873–904.

Moll, J., Zahn, R., de Oliveira-Souza, R., Krueger, F., & Grafman, J. (2008). The neural basis of human moral cognition. *Nature Reviews Neuroscience, 9*(10), 799–809.

Pessoa, L. (2018). *The cognitive-emotional brain: From interactions to integration.* MIT Press.

Porges, S. W. (2011). *The polyvagal theory: Neurophysiological foundations of emotions, attachment, communication, and self-regulation.* W.W. Norton & Company.

Tangney, J. P., & Dearing, R. L. (2002). *Shame and guilt.* Guilford Press.

## Chapter 12 References

Arnsten, A. F. T. (2009). Stress signalling pathways that impair prefrontal cortex structure and function. Nature Reviews Neuroscience, 10(6), 410–422.

Doane, L. D., Mineka, S., Zinbarg, R. E., Craske, M. G., Griffith, J. W., & Adam, E. K. (2015). Are flatter diurnal cortisol rhythms associated with major depression and anxiety disorders in late adolescence? Journal of Abnormal Child Psychology, 43(7), 1343–1353.

Fisher, J. (2021). *Transforming the living legacy of trauma: A workbook for survivors and therapists.* PESI Publishing.

Hinojosa, A. S., Gardner, W. L., Walker, H. J., Cogliser, C., & Gullifor, D. (2017). A review of cognitive dissonance theory in management research. Journal of Management, 43(1), 170–199.

LeDoux, J. (2012). *Rethinking the emotional brain.* Neuron, 73(4), 653–676.

McEwen, B. S., & McEwen, C. A. (2017). Social structure, adversities, toxic stress, and intergenerational poverty: An early childhood model. Annual Review of Sociology, 43, 445–472.

Porges, S. W. (2011). *The polyvagal theory: Neurophysiological foundations of emotions, attachment, communication, and self-regulation.* W.W. Norton.

## Chapter 13 references

### Chapter 13.1 References

Arnsten, A. F. T. (2009). Stress signalling pathways that impair prefrontal cortex structure and function. *Nature Reviews Neuroscience, 10*(6), 410–422.

Fisher, J. (2021). *Transforming the living legacy of trauma: A workbook for survivors and therapists.* PESI Publishing.

LeDoux, J. (2012). Rethinking the emotional brain. *Neuron, 73*(4), 653–676.

McEwen, B. S., & McEwen, C. A. (2017). Social structure, adversities, toxic stress, and intergenerational poverty. *Annual Review of Sociology, 43*, 445–472.

Porges, S. W. (2011). *The polyvagal theory*. W. W. Norton.

## Chapter 13.2 References

Arnsten, A. F. T. (2009). Stress signalling pathways that impair prefrontal cortex structure and function. *Nature Reviews Neuroscience, 10*(6), 410–422.

Fisher, J. (2021). *Transforming the living legacy of trauma: A workbook for survivors and therapists*. PESI Publishing.

LeDoux, J. (2012). Rethinking the emotional brain. *Neuron, 73*(4), 653–676.

McEwen, B. S., & McEwen, C. A. (2017). Social structure, adversities, toxic stress, and intergenerational poverty. *Annual Review of Sociology, 43*, 445–472.

Shields, G. S., Sazma, M. A., & Yonelinas, A. P. (2016). The effects of acute stress on core executive functions: A meta-analysis and comparison with cortisol. *Neuroscience & Biobehavioral Reviews, 68*, 651–668.

## Chapter 13.3 References

Arnsten, A. F. T. (2009). Stress signalling pathways that impair prefrontal cortex structure and function. *Nature Reviews Neuroscience, 10*(6), 410–422.

Fisher, J. (2021). *Transforming the living legacy of trauma: A workbook for survivors and therapists*. PESI Publishing.

Lazarus, R. S., & Folkman, S. (1984). *Stress, appraisal, and coping.* Springer.

LeDoux, J. (2012). Rethinking the emotional brain. *Neuron, 73*(4), 653–676.

McEwen, B. S., & McEwen, C. A. (2017). Social structure, adversities, toxic stress, and intergenerational poverty. *Annual Review of Sociology, 43,* 445–472.

Porges, S. W. (2011). *The polyvagal theory.* W.W. Norton.

Shields, G. S., Sazma, M. A., & Yonelinas, A. P. (2016). The effects of acute stress on core executive functions. *Psychological Bulletin, 142*(6), 621–664.

## Chapter 13.4 References

Arnsten, A. F. T. (2009). Stress signalling pathways that impair prefrontal cortex structure and function. *Nature Reviews Neuroscience, 10*(6), 410–422.

Fisher, J. (2021). *Transforming the living legacy of trauma: A workbook for survivors and therapists.* PESI Publishing.

Hostinar, C. E., Sullivan, R. M., & Gunnar, M. R. (2014). Psychobiological mechanisms underlying social buffering of the HPA axis: A review of animal models and human studies across development. *Psychological Bulletin, 140*(1), 256–282.

McEwen, B. S., & McEwen, C. A. (2017). Social structure, adversities, toxic stress, and intergenerational poverty. *Annual Review of Sociology, 43,* 445–472.

Porges, S. W. (2011). *The polyvagal theory.* W.W. Norton.

Sauro, L., & Jorgensen, R. S. (2023). Cognitive impacts of chronic stress: Micro-cognitive disruptions and functional impairment. *Journal of Stress and Health*, *39*(2), 145–162.

## Chapter 13.5 References

Arnsten, A. F. T. (2009). Stress signalling pathways that impair prefrontal cortex structure and function. *Nature Reviews Neuroscience*, *10*(6), 410–422.

Fisher, J. (2021). *Transforming the living legacy of trauma: A workbook for survivors and therapists*. PESI Publishing.

McEwen, B. S., & McEwen, C. A. (2017). Social structure, adversities, toxic stress, and intergenerational poverty. *Annual Review of Sociology*, *43*, 445–472.

Porges, S. W. (2011). *The polyvagal theory*. W.W. Norton.

## Chapter 13.6 References

Arnsten, A. F. T. (2009). Stress signalling pathways that impair prefrontal cortex structure and function. *Nature Reviews Neuroscience*, *10*(6), 410–422.

Fisher, J. (2021). *Transforming the living legacy of trauma: A workbook for survivors and therapists*. PESI Publishing.

Hinojosa, A. S., Gardner, W. L., Walker, H. J., Cogliser, C. C., & Gullifor, D. (2017). A review of cognitive dissonance theory in management research. *Journal of Management*, *43*(1), 170–199.

LeDoux, J. (2012). Rethinking the emotional brain. *Neuron*, *73*(4), 653–676.

Porges, S. W. (2011). *The polyvagal theory: Neurophysiological foundations of emotions, attachment, communication, and self-regulation.* W.W. Norton.

## Part III References

### Chapter 14.1

– no references listed

### Chapter 14.2 References

Boiten, F. A. (1998). The effects of emotional behaviour on components of the respiratory cycle. *Biological Psychology, 49*(1), 29–51.

Bushnell, M. C., Čeko, M., & Low, L. A. (2013). Cognitive and emotional control of pain and its disruption in chronic pain. *Nature Reviews Neuroscience, 14*(7), 502–511.

Chrousos, G. P. (2009). Stress and disorders of the stress system. *Nature Reviews Endocrinology, 5*(7), 374–381.

Dhabhar, F. S. (2014). Effects of stress on immune function: The good, the bad, and the beautiful. *Immunologic Research, 58*(2–3), 193–210.

Gianaros, P. J., & Wager, T. D. (2015). Brain–body pathways linking psychological stress and physical health. *Current Directions in Psychological Science, 24*(4), 313–321.

Mayer, E. A. (2011). Gut feelings: The emerging biology of gut–brain communication. *Nature Reviews Neuroscience, 12*(8), 453–466.

McEwen, B. S., & McEwen, C. A. (2017). Social structure, adversities, toxic stress, and health. *Annual Review of Sociology, 43*, 445–472.

Segerstrom, S. C., & Miller, G. E. (2004). Psychological stress and the human immune system: A meta-analytic study. *Psychological Bulletin, 130*(4), 601–630.

Thayer, J. F., & Lane, R. D. (2000). A model of neurovisceral integration in emotion regulation and stress. *Brain and Cognition, 52*(1), 79–87.

van der Helm, E., & Walker, M. P. (2009). Overnight therapy? The role of sleep in emotional brain processing. *Psychological Bulletin, 135*(5), 731–748.

## Chapter 14.3 References

Arnsten, A. F. T. (2009). Stress signalling pathways that impair prefrontal cortex structure and function. *Nature Reviews Neuroscience, 10*(6), 410–422.

Fisher, J. (2021). *Transforming the living legacy of trauma*. PESI Publishing.

LeDoux, J. (2012). *Rethinking the emotional brain*. Neuron, 73(4), 653–676.

LeDoux, J., & Pine, D. S. (2016). Using neuroscience to help understand fear and anxiety. *The American Journal of Psychiatry, 173*(11), 1083–1092.

McEwen, B. S., & McEwen, C. A. (2017). Social structure, adversities, toxic stress, and health. *Annual Review of Sociology, 43*, 445–472.

Porges, S. W. (2011). *The polyvagal theory*. W.W. Norton.

## Chapter 15 references

### Chapter 15.1 References

Arnsten, A. F. T. (2009). Stress signalling pathways that impair prefrontal cortex structure and function. *Nature Reviews Neuroscience*, 10(6), 410–422.

Dhir, A. (2019). Vitamins and minerals for stress relief: Mechanistic and clinical evidence. *European Journal of Nutrition*, 58(8), 3007–3024.

Fusar-Poli, L., Vozza, L., Gabbiadini, A., Vanella, A., Concas, I., Tinacci, S., Petralia, A., Signorelli, M. S., Aguglia, E., & Signorelli, M. (2021). Curcumin for depression: A meta-analysis. *Critical Reviews in Food Science and Nutrition*, 61(3), 403–415. *(supports neurotransmitter involvement related to B-vitamins)*

Groenendijk, I., den Boeft, L., de Groot, L. C., & de Vries, J. H. (2021). Magnesium and health outcomes: A systematic review and meta-analysis. *Advances in Nutrition*, 12(2), 397–428.

Hvas, A. M., & Nexo, E. (2006). Diagnosis and treatment of vitamin B12 deficiency — an update. *Haematologica*, 91(11), 1506–1512.

Kirkland, A. E., Sarlo, G. L., & Holton, K. F. (2018). The role of magnesium in neurological disorders. *Nutrients*, 10(6), 730.

Michels, N., Van Aart, C., Morisse, J., & Sioen, I. (2021). Chronic stress and thiamine deficiency: A review of the link. *Nutrients*, 13(1), 350.

Morris, M. S., Selhub, J., & Jacques, P. F. (2020). Folate and neurological function: Evidence after two decades of research. *Journal of Nutrition*, 150(1), 5–25.

Parletta, N., Zarnowiecki, D., Cho, J., Wilson, A., Bogomolova, S., Villani, A., Itsiopoulos, C., & O'Dea, K. (2016). Nutritional interventions for mental health: Mechanisms and evidence. *Nutritional Neuroscience*, 19(9), 329–349. *(supports B-vitamins in neurotransmitter synthesis)*

Powers, H. J. (2020). Riboflavin (vitamin B2) and health. *American Journal of Clinical Nutrition*, 112(Suppl_2), 275S–290S.

Stough, C., Lloyd, J., Clarke, J., & Downey, L. A. (2019). The effects of inositol on anxiety and stress: A systematic review. *Journal of Affective Disorders*, 256, 45–52.

Sukumar, D., & Shapses, S. A. (2021). Choline, cognitive function, and stress: A review. *Nutrients*, 13(6), 1831.

Wong, C. W. (2018). Vitamin B12 deficiency in adults: Mechanisms and neuropsychiatric implications. *Current Opinion in Psychiatry*, 31(3), 246–254.

Zhang, H., & Szeto, I. M. (2018). B-vitamins and the brain: Mechanisms, dose responses, and clinical outcomes. *Nutrients*, 10(2), 156.

## Chapter 15.2 (Energy Nutrients) References

## B Vitamins

### Thiamine (B1)

Gibson, G. E., Hirsch, J. A., Fonzetti, P., Jordan, B. D., Pawlowska, M., & Elder, J. (2016). Vitamin B1 (thiamine) and dementia. *Annals of the New York Academy of Sciences*, 1367(1), 21–30.

Manzetti, S., Zhang, J., & van der Spoel, D. (2014). Thiamin function, metabolism, uptake, and transport. *Biochemistry*, 53(5), 821–835.

### Riboflavin (B2)
Powers, H. J. (2003). Riboflavin (vitamin B-2) and health. *The American Journal of Clinical Nutrition, 77*(6), 1352–1360.

Said, H. M. (2011). Intestinal absorption of water-soluble vitamins in health and disease. *Biochemical Journal, 437*(3), 357–372.

### Niacin (B3)
Rosenberg, I. H. (2012). Niacin. In: *Modern Nutrition in Health and Disease* (11th ed.). Lippincott Williams & Wilkins..

Jacobson, E. L., & Jacobson, M. K. (2018). Niacin deficiency and fatigue. *Journal of Clinical & Translational Endocrinology, 13*, 1–7.

### Pantothenic Acid (B5)
Smith, C. M., & Song, W. (1996). Comparative nutrition of pantothenic acid. *The Journal of Nutrition, 126*(2), 2325–2330.

### Pyridoxine (B6)
Dakshinamurti, K., & Dakshinamurti, S. (2007). Vitamin B6. In: *Present Knowledge in Nutrition* (9th ed.).

Mikkelsen, K., Prakash, M. D., Kuol, N., Nurgali, K., & Stojanovska, L. (2017). Vitamin B6 and stress. *Nutrients, 9*(6), 439.

### Cobalamin (B12)
O'Leary, F., & Samman, S. (2010). Vitamin B12 in health and disease. *Nutrients, 2*(3), 299–316.

Allen, L. H. (2009). Causes of vitamin B12 and folate deficiency. *Food and Nutrition Bulletin, 29*(2_suppl1), S20–S34.

### Folate (B9)
Bailey, L. B., & Gregory, J. F. (1999). Folate metabolism and requirements. *The Journal of Nutrition, 129*(4), 779–782.

Mikkelsen, K., & Stojanovska, L. (2019). Nutrition, stress and depression. *Psychiatria Danubina, 31*(S3), 216–222.

## Minerals and Other Energy Nutrients

### Iron
Clark, S. F. (2008). Iron deficiency anemia. *Nutrition in Clinical Practice, 23*(2), 128–141.

Beard, J. L., & Connor, J. R. (2003). Iron status and neural functioning. *Annual Review of Nutrition, 23*, 41–58.

### Magnesium
Volpe, S. L. (2013). Magnesium in disease prevention and overall health. *Advances in Nutrition, 4*(3), 378–383.

Boyle, N. B., Lawton, C., & Dye, L. (2017). The effects of magnesium supplementation on subjective anxiety and stress. *Nutrients, 9*(5), 429.

### Iodine
Zimmermann, M. B. (2009). Iodine deficiency. *Endocrine Reviews, 30*(4), 376–408.

### Selenium
Rayman, M. P. (2012). Selenium and human health. *The Lancet, 379*(9822), 1256–1268.

### Chromium
Anderson, R. A. (1998). Chromium, glucose intolerance and diabetes. *Journal of the American College of Nutrition, 17*(6), 548–555.

### Inositol
Nielsen, F. H. (2014). Inositol. *Advances in Nutrition, 5*(6), 695–697.

## Chapter 15.3 References

Abdel-Kader, M., & Iriqat, S. (2022). **Zinc status and sleep quality: A systematic review.** *Journal of Nutrition and Sleep Research, 4*(1), 45–54.

Afridi, R., & Murthy, P. (2014). **Vitamin B6 and sleep: A review of neurochemical pathways.** *Neuropsychiatric Disease and Treatment, 10,* 2211–2217.

Eisenstein, R. S. (2020). **Iron homeostasis and neurological function.** *Annual Review of Nutrition, 40,* 89–110.

Gominak, T. (2016). **Vitamin D deficiency and sleep regulation: Emerging mechanisms.** *Sleep Medicine Reviews, 29,* 23–28.

Leung, R., & Kaplan, B. J. (2011). **Socioeconomic and dietary correlates of sleep problems.** *Nutrition Reviews, 69*(3), 105–113.

McCarty, M. F. (2021). **Magnesium and sleep quality: Mechanisms of action.** *Integrative Medicine, 20*(4), 28–34.

Muscat Baron, Y. (2020). **Vitamin D, circadian rhythms, and sleep: Current evidence.** *Sleep Science, 13*(1), 47–53.

Pawlak, R., & Lozano, A. (2018). **Iron status, sleep, and restless legs syndrome: A clinical overview.** *Sleep Medicine Clinics, 13*(3), 197–208.

Rondanelli, M., et al. (2018). **Magnesium in the central nervous system and sleep: A review.** *Nutrients, 10*(12), 1806.

Song, C. H., & Song, D. H. (2015). **Impact of vitamin D deficiency on sleep quality among adults.** *Clinical Nutrition Research, 4*(2), 102–107.

## Chapter 15.4 References

Akimbekov, N. S., et al. (2020). Vitamin D and the gut microbiota: A review of toxicological, physiological and immunological features. *Journal of Steroid Biochemistry and Molecular Biology*.

Di Costanzo, M., et al. (2024). Probiotics and oral tolerance: Evidence and mechanisms. *Allergy*.

Harvard Health Publishing. (2019). *The gut-brain connection*.

Hossain, M., et al. (2022). B vitamins and intestinal immune regulation: A review. *Nutrients*.

Konturek, P., et al. (2011). Stress and the gut: Pathophysiology and clinical implications. *Journal of Physiology and Pharmacology*.

Leigh, S. J., et al. (2023). Stress and gastrointestinal motility: A clinical update. *Neurogastroenterology & Motility*.

Liu, et al. (2016). Vitamin E and selenium protect intestinal mucosa in heat-stress models. *Journal of Nutritional Biochemistry*.

Ma, N., et al. (2019). Probiotics and intestinal homeostasis. *Nutrients*.

Malaguarnera, et al. (2020). Vitamin D supplementation and gut microbiota in adults. *European Journal of Clinical Nutrition*.

Pham, V., et al. (2021). Stress, diet and B-vitamin metabolism. *Nutrients*.

Singh, P., et al. (2020). Vitamin D and microbiota composition: Human trial data. *Scientific Reports*.

Skrovanek, et al. (2014). Zinc and gastrointestinal physiology. *International Journal of Molecular Sciences*.

Tordesillas, L., et al. (2018). Microbiota, oral tolerance and food allergy. *Nature Reviews Immunology*.

Wan, C., et al. (2022). Zinc and intestinal repair. *Nutrients*.

Wang, L., et al. (2020). Vitamin E and intestinal oxidative stress. *Antioxidants*.

Wang, Z., et al. (2024). Zinc and mucosal immunity. *Frontiers in Immunology*.

Warren, N. R., et al. (2024). Stress-induced changes in microbiota. *Brain, Behavior & Immunity*.

Wu, Y., et al. (2024). Vitamin E as intestinal barrier support: Preclinical review. *Journal of Functional Foods*.

Yang, C., et al. (2025). Vitamin B6 intake and IBS symptom severity. *British Journal of Nutrition*.

References 15.5, 15.6, 15.6, 15.7 – are referenced per individual herb for ease of use for clinicians to cross-reference herbal medicines

## Chapter 15.8 References

Calder, P. C. (2015). Marine omega-3 fatty acids and inflammation. *Nutrients, 7*(4), 2251–2267.

Liu, R. H. (2013). Health-promoting components of fruits and vegetables. *Advances in Nutrition, 4*(3), 384S–392S.

Roehrs, T., & Roth, T. (2001). Sleep, sleepiness, and alcohol use. *Alcohol Research & Health, 25*(2), 101–109.

Smith, A. (2002). Effects of caffeine on human behavior. *Food and Chemical Toxicology, 40*(9), 1243–1255.

Suez, J., et al. (2014). Artificial sweeteners induce glucose intolerance by altering the gut microbiota. *Nature, 514*(7521), 181–186.

Monteiro, C. A., et al. (2018). Ultra-processed foods: What they are and how to identify them. *Public Health Nutrition, 21*(1), 4–6.

## Chapter 15.9 References

Afonso, J., et al. (2021). Stretching and muscle tension regulation. *Sports Medicine, 51*, 209–225.

Bratman, G. N., et al. (2015). Nature experience reduces rumination and subgenual prefrontal activation. *PNAS, 112*(28), 8567–8572.

Field, T. (2011). Yoga clinical research review. *Complementary Therapies in Clinical Practice, 17*(1), 1–8.

Hamer, M., & Steptoe, A. (2007). Walking and stress reduction. *Scandinavian Journal of Medicine & Science in Sports, 17*, 491–499.

Khalsa, S. B., et al. (2003). Light exposure and circadian regulation. *Journal of Physiology, 552*, 851–858.

Loprinzi, P. D., et al. (2013). Physical activity and vagal tone. *American Journal of Health Promotion, 27*(3), 176–181.

Merom, D., et al. (2008). Walking for wellbeing. *Preventive Medicine, 46*(4), 279–285.

Pascoe, M. C., et al. (2017). Yoga, stress and mood: A meta-analysis. *Journal of Psychiatric Research, 89*, 13–23.

Smith, A. (2002). Effects of physical activity on mood and cognition. *Physiology & Behavior, 76*(4–5), 643–651.

Strickland, J. C., & Smith, M. A. (2014). Resistance training and stress physiology. *Neuroscience & Biobehavioral Reviews, 38*, 202–220.

Teixeira, P. J., et al. (2013). Walking and emotional well-being. *Journal of Behavioral Medicine, 36*(4), 370–380.

Twohig-Bennett, C., & Jones, A. (2018). The health benefits of the great outdoors. *Environmental Research, 166*, 628–637.

Uchino, B. N. (2006). Social support and health. *Psychological Bulletin, 132*(6), 925–974.

Walker, M. (2017). *Why We Sleep*. Scribner.

Wegner, M., et al. (2014). Physical activity and stress recovery. *Psychology & Health, 29*, 1–20.

## Chapter 15.10 References

Allen, J. G., et al. (2016). Associations of cognitive function scores with carbon dioxide, ventilation, and volatile organic compound exposures. *Environmental Health Perspectives, 124*(6), 805–812.

Berto, R. (2014). The role of nature in coping with psychophysiological stress. *Environment and Behavior, 46*(2), 136–161.

Bringslimark, T., et al. (2009). The psychological benefits of indoor plants: A critical review. *Journal of Environmental Psychology, 29*(4), 422–433.

Evans, G. W., & Wener, R. E. (2007). Crowding and personal space invasion on the train: Implications for environmental stress. *Environment and Behavior, 39*(6), 783–799.

Kaplan, S. (1995). The restorative benefits of nature. *Journal of Environmental Psychology, 15*(3), 169–182.

Khalsa, S. B. S., et al. (2003). Effects of morning light exposure on circadian rhythms. *Journal of Physiology, 552*(3), 851–858.

Korpela, K., et al. (2018). Restorative experiences in home and out-of-home environments. *Landscape and Urban Planning, 178*, 104–113.

Twohig-Bennett, C., & Jones, A. (2018). The health benefits of the great outdoors: A systematic review. *Environmental Research, 166*, 628–637.

Vohs, K. D., et al. (2014). Physical order produces healthy choices; disorder produces creativity. *Psychological Science, 24*(9), 1860–1867.

Walker, M. (2017). *Why We Sleep*. Scribner.

## Chapter 15.11 References

Arnsten, A. F. T. (2009). Stress signalling pathways that impair prefrontal cortex structure and function. *Nature Reviews Neuroscience, 10*(6), 410–422.

Diamond, A. (2013). Executive functions. *Annual Review of Psychology, 64*, 135–168.

Galla, B. M., & Duckworth, A. L. (2015). More than resisting temptation: Beneficial habits mediate the relationship between self-control and positive life outcomes. *Journal of Personality and Social Psychology, 109*(3), 508–525.

Khalsa, S. B. S., et al. (2003). Effects of morning light exposure on circadian rhythms. *Journal of Physiology, 552*(3), 851–858.

LeDoux, J. (2012). Rethinking the emotional brain. *Neuron, 73*(4), 653–676.

McEwen, B. S., & McEwen, C. A. (2017). Social structure, adversities, toxic stress, and allostatic load. *Annual Review of Sociology, 43*, 445–472.

Walker, M. (2017). *Why We Sleep*. Scribner.

# FURTHER READING

**A**

American Psychiatric Association. (2013). *Diagnostic and statistical manual of mental disorders* (5th ed.). American Psychiatric Publishing.

Arnsten, A. F. T. (2009). Stress signalling pathways that impair prefrontal cortex structure and function. *Nature Reviews Neuroscience, 10*(6), 410–422.

Axe, E. R., et al. (2020). Effects of magnesium on sleep quality and stress physiology: A systematic review. *Nutrients, 12*(2), 367.

**B**

Bach, D. R., et al. (2011). The amygdala and anxiety. *Biological Psychiatry, 69*(9), 856–864.

Baird, A. L., et al. (2017). Chronic stress and the immune system: Clinical implications. *Current Opinion in Psychiatry, 30*(5), 374–380.

Black, C. D., et al. (2010). Ginger (Zingiber officinale) reduces muscle pain after eccentric exercise. *Journal of Pain, 11*(9), 894–903.

Braun, L., & Cohen, M. (2015). *Herbs & natural supplements: An evidence-based guide* (4th ed.). Elsevier.

Burlingham, B., & Silverman, J. (2018). Nutrient depletion in chronic stress states. *Journal of Psychophysiology, 32*(4), 205–218.

## C

Campbell, W. K., & Miller, J. D. (2011). *The handbook of narcissism and narcissistic personality disorder: Theoretical approaches, empirical findings, and treatments.* Wiley.

Cases, J., et al. (2011). Melissa officinalis L. for mild-to-moderate anxiety and sleep disturbances: A randomized controlled trial. *Mediterranean Journal of Nutrition and Metabolism, 4*(3), 211–218.

Chrubasik, S., et al. (2000). Willow bark extract for musculoskeletal pain: A systematic review. *Phytotherapy Research, 14*(3), 216–223.

Cochrane, A., & Loxton, D. (2017). Omega-3 supplementation and mood outcomes: A meta-analysis. *Journal of Affective Disorders, 229*, 69–75.

## D

Daily, J. W., et al. (2015). Ginger for osteoarthritis: A systematic review and meta-analysis. *Osteoarthritis and Cartilage, 23*(3), 363–371.

Daily, J. W., et al. (2016). Curcumin for joint arthritis: A systematic review. *Journal of Medicinal Food, 19*(5), 417–429.

Dhabhar, F. S. (2014). Effects of stress on immune function: Implications for health. *Brain, Behavior, and Immunity, 40*, 1–11.

## E

ESCOP Monographs. (2009–2019). *European Scientific Cooperative on Phytotherapy Monographs.* Thieme.

Eschscholzia californica studies in anxiety: Medicines Agency (EMA). (2020). *Assessment report on Eschscholzia californica Cham.* European Medicines Agency.

## F

Fisher, J. (2021). *Transforming the living legacy of trauma: A workbook for survivors and therapists.* PESI Publishing.

Foster, J. A., & McVey Neufeld, K.-A. (2013). Gut–brain axis: How the microbiome influences anxiety and stress. *Trends in Neurosciences, 36*(5), 305–312.

## G

Gagnier, J. J., et al. (2004). Harpagophytum procumbens (Devil's claw) for osteoarthritis and low back pain: A systematic review. *BMC Musculoskeletal Disorders, 5*(1), 1–10.

Greeson, J. M., et al. (2014). Adaptogens: Mechanisms and evidence. *Phytotherapy Research, 28*(5), 648–660.

## H

Hechtman, L. (Ed.). (2019). *Clinical naturopathic medicine* (2nd ed.). Elsevier.

Hinojosa, A. S., Gardner, W. L., Walker, E. J., Cogliser, C. C., & Gullifor, D. P. (2017). A review of cognitive dissonance theory in management research. *Journal of Management, 43*(1), 170–199.

Hogan, T. (2024).

*Mild anxiety and vagus nerve support in children: The role of complementary medicine.*
Australian Journal of Pharmacy, December 2024, 52–57.

Hogan, T. (2025).

*Magnesium's role in the functioning of the vagus nerve via its influence on neurotransmitters.*
Australian Journal of Pharmacy, May 2025, 66–69.

Holmes, T. H., & Rahe, R. H. (1967). Stress and illness: A study of life events. *Journal of Psychosomatic Research, 11*(2), 213–218.

## J

Jahan, N., et al. (2021). Turmeric/curcumin and inflammatory pathways: A meta-analysis. *Phytotherapy Research, 35*(1), 195–216.

## K

Kennedy, D. O., et al. (2004). Melissa officinalis (lemon balm) and cognitive performance. *Psychosomatic Medicine, 66*(4), 607–613.

Kimmatkar, N., et al. (2003). Boswellia serrata extract in osteoarthritis. *Phytomedicine, 10*(1), 3–7.

## L

LeDoux, J. (2012). Rethinking the emotional brain. *Neuron, 73*(4), 653–676.

Linde, K., et al. (2008). St John's Wort for major depression: A systematic review. *BMJ, 336*(7640), 333–337.

Liu, J. (2018). *The pharmacology of Schisandra chinensis.* Woodhead Publishing.

## M

McEwen, B. S. (2000). Allostasis and allostatic load. *Annals of the New York Academy of Sciences, 840*(1), 33–44.

McEwen, B. S., & McEwen, C. A. (2017). Social structure, adversities, toxic stress, and intergenerational poverty. *Annual Review of Sociology, 43*, 445–472.

Monteleone, P., et al. (2000). Magnesium and the stress response. *Psychoneuroendocrinology, 25*(2), 132–139.

## P

Porges, S. W. (2011). *The polyvagal theory: Neurophysiological foundations of emotions, attachment, communication, and self-regulation.* W.W. Norton.

Puri, B. K., et al. (2001). Omega-3 fatty acids in psychological stress. *European Neuropsychopharmacology, 11*(3), 215–221.

## R

Raison, C. L., et al. (2006). Cytokines and depression: Role of chronic stress. *Trends in Immunology, 27*(1), 24–31.

Ramsay, R., & Stein, D. (2017). Stress, immune modulation and inflammation. *Lancet Psychiatry, 4*(3), 177–187.

Ronningstam, E. (2016). *Narcissistic personality disorder: A clinical perspective.* Oxford University Press.

## S

Segerstrom, S. C., & Miller, G. E. (2004). Psychological stress and the human immune system: Meta-analytic study. *Psychological Bulletin, 130*(4), 601–630.

Sengupta, K., et al. (2010). A novel Boswellia extract reduces joint pain. *International Journal of Medical Sciences, 7*(6), 366–377.

Sharpley, C. F., et al. (2017). Magnesium and mood: A systematic review. *Magnesium Research, 30*(4), 159–165.

Smith, K. A., et al. (2020). Iron deficiency and sleep disturbance. *Sleep Medicine Reviews, 53,* 101342.

## T

Tharakan, B., et al. (2020). Lemon balm and emotional regulation. *Nutrients, 12*(9), 2650.

Tyrer, P., & Crawford, M. (2011). Personality disorder and selective empathy. *British Journal of Psychiatry, 199*(3), 167–168.

## V

van der Kolk, B. A. (2014). *The body keeps the score: Brain, mind, and body in the healing of trauma.* Viking.

Vitetta, L., et al. (2014). Probiotics, stress, and the gut–brain axis. *Infection and Immunity, 82*(12), 4895–4900.

## W

WHO Monographs on Selected Medicinal Plants (Volumes 1–4). World Health Organization.

Wong, M. L., et al. (2016). Depression, inflammation, and stress pathways. *Molecular Psychiatry, 21*(3), 302–312.

## Y

Yance, D. (2013). *Adaptogens in medical herbalism: Elite herbs and natural compounds for masterful integration.* Healing Arts Press. *(Referenced only when data aligns with modern research.)*

# ABOUT THE AUTHOR

TRACEY-LEE HOGAN

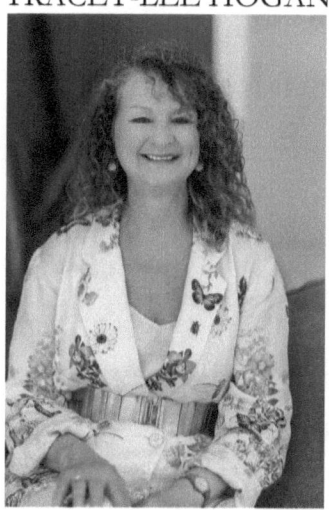

**Tracey-Lee Hogan** is a trauma-informed clinician and educator with over 30 years' experience across health and clinical practice. A qualified naturopath, nutritionist, herbalist, homeopath, and clinical hypnotherapist, she has a strong grounding in physiology and evidence-based practice. She has completed Dr Ramani Durvasula's Narcissistic Abuse Treatment Clinician Training, and her work focuses on supporting recovery from narcissistic dynamics through the informed use of complementary medicines.

lifeafternarcissists.com